Diabetes

Fight It
with
the Blood
Type Diet®

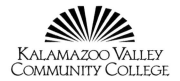

Also by Dr. Peter J. D'Adamo with Catherine Whitney

Eat Right 4 Your Type: The Individualized Diet Solution to Staying Healthy, Living Longer, and Achieving Your Ideal Weight

Cook Right 4 Your Type: The Practical Kitchen Companion to Eat Right 4 Your Type

Live Right 4 Your Type: The Individualized Prescription for Maximizing Health, Metabolism, and Vitality in Every Stage of Your Life

Eat Right 4 Your Baby: The Individualized Guide to Fertility and Maximum Health During Pregnancy, Nursing, and Your Baby's First Year

Eat Right 4 Your Type Complete Blood Type Encyclopedia

Blood Type O: Food, Beverage and Supplement Lists

Blood Type A: Food, Beverage and Supplement Lists

Blood Type B: Food, Beverage and Supplement Lists

Blood Type AB: Food, Beverage and Supplement Lists

DR. PETER J. D'ADAMO

WITH CATHERINE WHITNEY

Dr. Peter J. D'Adamo's

Eat Right for Your Type

Health Library

Diabetes

Fight It
with
the Blood
Type Diet®

G. P. PUTNAM'S SONS

NEW YORK

G. P. Putnam's Sons
Publishers Since 1838
a member of
Penguin Group (USA) Inc.
375 Hudson Street
New York, NY 10014

Library of Congress Cataloging-in-Publication Data

D'Adamo, Peter.
Diabetes : fight it with the blood type diet / Peter J. D'Adamo
with Catherine Whitney.
p.   cm.—(Dr. Peter J. D'Adamo's eat right 4 your type health library)
Includes index.
ISBN 0-399-15102-8
1. Diabetes—Diet therapy.   2. Blood groups.   I. Whitney,
Catherine (Catherine A.).   II. Title.   III. Series.
RC662.D33   2004   2003058455
616.4'620654—dc22

Printed in the United States of America
1   3   5   7   9   10   8   6   4   2

This book is printed on acid-free paper. ∞

DEDICATED TO MY PATIENTS,
WHOSE COURAGE AND DETERMINATION
IS A DAILY INSPIRATION

Acknowledgments

THIS BOOK OFFERS THE BEST THAT NATUROPATHIC MEDICINE and blood type science have to offer in the management of diabetes. It has been a collaborative process, and I want to express my deep thanks to the people who have been involved in its creation.

I am most grateful to Martha Mosko D'Adamo, not only my partner in life and in parenting, but also my partner in bringing the valuable wisdom about blood type to the world. Martha daily provides love, support, insight, and inspiration to all of my endeavors.

Catherine Whitney, my writer, and her partner, Paul Krafin, are invaluable word masters who have once again captured exactly the right tone in tackling this complex topic.

My literary agent and friend, Janis Vallely, always takes time to listen and advise. Her quiet guidance and personal support make the work possible.

I would also like to acknowledge others who have made significant contributions to this book: my colleague Bronner Handwerger, N.D., whose research and clinical abilities helped make this book comprehensive and practical; John Harris, whose knowledge and support have been invaluable; Heidi Merritt, who continues to make an important contribution to the work; and Jane Dystel, Catherine's literary agent.

Amy Hertz, my editor at Riverhead/Putnam, has been the force behind the success of all the blood type books, and she continues to guide my work with dedication and skill.

As always, I am extremely grateful to the wonderful staff at Riverhead Books and Putnam. They have been tireless and enthusiastic, and their efforts have made it possible to continue bringing this important work to the market.

PETER J. D'ADAMO, N.D.

Contents

Diabetes

Fight It
with
the Blood
Type Diet®

New Tools to Fight Diabetes

E VERYONE CAN BENEFIT FROM FOLLOWING THE BLOOD TYPE
Diet. You don't have to be sick to see the effects. But most of the
people who come to my clinic or contact my Web site are dealing with
a serious chronic disease or have received a distressing medical diagnosis. They want to know how they can hone the general guidelines
of the Blood Type Diet to target their illness. Dr. Peter J. D'Adamo's
Eat Right 4 (for) Your Type Health Library has been introduced with
these people in mind.

Diabetes: Fight It with the Blood Type Diet allows you to take full advantage of the medicinal benefits of eating and living according to your
blood type. If you think of the standard Blood Type Diet as the foun-
dation, the guidelines in this book provide a more targeted overlay for
people who have diabetes, pre-diabetes, hypoglycemia, or hyperglycemia. These dietary and lifestyle adaptations, individualized by
blood type, supply additional ammunition to your disease-fighting ar-
senal. Specifically, they can help you control your blood sugar, achieve
a healthy weight, improve your metabolic fitness, increase your energy

and well-being, and reduce or eliminate the need for medications that treat type 2 diabetes.

Here's what you'll find that's new:

- A disease-fighting category of blood type–specific food values, the **Super Beneficials,** emphasizing foods that have medicinal properties in regulating blood sugar, reducing LDL cholesterol and triglyceride levels, normalizing blood pressure and thyroid function, and improving overall metabolic health.
- A disease-specific breakdown of the **Neutral** category to limit foods that are known to have less nutritional value, or that may exacerbate your condition. Foods designated **Neutral: Allowed Infrequently** should be minimized or avoided by people who are diabetic or pre-diabetic. That means consuming them no more than once or twice a month. To increase your level of compliance, avoid them altogether.
- Detailed Supplement Protocols for each blood type that are calibrated to support you at every stage. They include a **Pre-Diabetes/Metabolic Enhancement Protocol,** and three adjunct protocols for **Type 1 Diabetes, Type 2 Diabetes,** and **Diabetic Complications.**
- A **4-Week Plan** for getting started that emphasizes what you can do immediately to improve your blood sugar regulation and start feeling better right away.
- Plus: many strategies for success, quizzes, and checklists, and answers to the questions most frequently asked about diabetes at my clinic.

The science of blood type continues to provide important clues to the biological and genetic mechanisms that control health and disease. In more than twenty-five years of research and clinical practice, I have successfully treated thousands of patients with diabetes and related metabolic conditions, using the Blood Type Diet. Increasingly, medical doctors and naturopaths throughout the world are applying the blood type principles in their practices with remarkable results.

I urge you to talk to your physician about the benefits of incorporating individualized, blood type–specific diet, exercise, and lifestyle strategies into your current plan. I am confident that using the guidelines in this book will start you on the road to health. Take the step now, and be true to your type.

What's Your Blood Type– Diabetes Risk?

Blood Type O Quiz
Are You Diabetes-Prone?

General Factors

The following factors are known to contribute to an individual's overall diabetes risk. Answer yes or no to each question.

1. Does a parent or sibling of yours have diabetes? ☐ yes ☐ no
2. Is your racial or ethnic background African-American, Hispanic, or Native American? ☐ yes ☐ no
3. Are you more than 20% overweight? ☐ yes ☐ no
4. Do you have high blood pressure? ☐ yes ☐ no
5. Do you have high cholesterol (overall above 200 and HDL under 45 mg/dL for men and 55 mg/dL for women)? ☐ yes ☐ no
6. Do you have a triglyceride level over 150 mg/dL? ☐ yes ☐ no
7. Are you 50 years old or older? ☐ yes ☐ no
8. Do you have a history of heavy alcohol use? ☐ yes ☐ no

9. Do you smoke?   ☐ yes ☐ no
10. (Women) Did you have gestational diabetes
    during pregnancy or deliver a child who
    weighed 9 pounds or more?   ☐ yes ☐ no
11. Do you suffer from an autoimmune disease?   ☐ yes ☐ no

Blood Type O–Specific Factors
The following factors are known to specifically influence Blood Type O's risk for obesity, insulin resistance, and diabetes. Answer yes or no to each question.

1. Do you consume a high-carbohydrate,
   low-protein diet?   ☐ yes ☐ no
2. Do you have a history of following very
   low-calorie "starvation" diets?   ☐ yes ☐ no
3. Have you been a "yo-yo" dieter?   ☐ yes ☐ no
4. Do you often skip meals?   ☐ yes ☐ no
5. Do you lead a sedentary lifestyle that includes
   little aerobic exercise?   ☐ yes ☐ no
6. Do you eat wheat every day?   ☐ yes ☐ no
7. Do you regularly consume refined sugars?   ☐ yes ☐ no
8. Is your diet low in fiber (less than 3–4 servings
   per day)?   ☐ yes ☐ no
9. Do you need stimulants (coffee, chocolate,
   cigarettes, etc.) to keep you going?   ☐ yes ☐ no

Scoring: Add the number of "yes" responses in each list. Your score is based on the total:

12–20: High Risk You are almost certainly heading toward type 2 diabetes (if you don't already have it). You need to act now to address the factors you can control. Review the items marked "yes." Some, such as your age, ethnicity, and family history, are beyond your control. However, your high score indicates that there are major areas that you can change.

8–11: Moderate Risk If you make some changes now, you can still prevent diabetes. Review the items marked "yes," paying special attention to those related to diet, exercise, and lifestyle, to determine the actions you must take.

0–7: Low Risk Your risk is not severe. Keep it that way by following the Blood Type O Diet and lifestyle plan.

Blood Type A Quiz
Are You Diabetes-Prone?

General Factors

The following factors are known to contribute to an individual's overall diabetes risk. Answer yes or no to each question.

1. Does a parent or sibling of yours have diabetes? ☐ yes ☐ no
2. Is your racial or ethnic background African-American, Hispanic, or Native American? ☐ yes ☐ no
3. Are you more than 20% overweight? ☐ yes ☐ no
4. Do you have high blood pressure? ☐ yes ☐ no
5. Do you have high cholesterol (overall above 200 and HDL under 45 mg/dL for men and 55 mg/dL for women)? ☐ yes ☐ no
6. Do you have a triglyceride level over 150 mg/dL? ☐ yes ☐ no
7. Are you 50 years old or older? ☐ yes ☐ no
8. Do you have a history of heavy alcohol use? ☐ yes ☐ no
9. Do you smoke? ☐ yes ☐ no
10. (Women) Did you have gestational diabetes during pregnancy or deliver a child who weighed 9 pounds or more? ☐ yes ☐ no
11. Do you suffer from an autoimmune disease? ☐ yes ☐ no

Blood Type A–Specific Factors

The following factors are known to specifically influence Blood Type A's risk for obesity, insulin resistance, and diabetes. Answer yes or no to each question.

1. Do you consume a high-protein, high-fat diet? ☐ yes ☐ no
2. Do you have a history of following very
   low-calorie "starvation" diets? ☐ yes ☐ no
3. Are you experiencing high stress levels? ☐ yes ☐ no
4. Do you frequently experience anxiety,
   sleep disruptions, and/or fatigue? ☐ yes ☐ no
5. Do you often skip meals? ☐ yes ☐ no
6. Do you avoid exercise, even stretching or yoga? ☐ yes ☐ no
7. Do you eat meat every day? ☐ yes ☐ no
8. Do you regularly consume refined sugars? ☐ yes ☐ no
9. Is your diet low in fiber (less than 3–4 servings
   per day)? ☐ yes ☐ no

Scoring: Add the number of "yes" responses in each list. Your score is based on the total:

12–20: High Risk You are almost certainly heading toward type 2 diabetes (if you don't already have it). You need to act now to address the factors you can control. Review the items marked "yes." Some, such as your age, ethnicity, and family history, are beyond your control. However, your high score indicates that there are major areas that you can change.

8–11: Moderate Risk If you make some changes now, you can still prevent diabetes. Review the items marked "yes," paying special attention to those related to diet, exercise, and lifestyle, to determine the actions you must take.

0–7: Low Risk Your risk is not severe. Keep it that way by following the Blood Type A Diet and lifestyle plan.

Blood Type B Quiz
Are You Diabetes-Prone?

General Factors

The following factors are known to contribute to an individual's overall diabetes risk. Answer yes or no to each question.

1. Does a parent or sibling of yours have diabetes? ☐ yes ☐ no
2. Is your racial or ethnic background African-American, Hispanic, or Native American? ☐ yes ☐ no
3. Are you more than 20% overweight? ☐ yes ☐ no
4. Do you have high blood pressure? ☐ yes ☐ no
5. Do you have high cholesterol (overall above 200 and HDL under 45 mg/dL for men and 55 mg/dL for women)? ☐ yes ☐ no
6. Do you have a triglyceride level over 150 mg/dL? ☐ yes ☐ no
7. Are you 50 years old or older? ☐ yes ☐ no
8. Do you have a history of heavy alcohol use? ☐ yes ☐ no
9. Do you smoke? ☐ yes ☐ no
10. (Women) Did you have gestational diabetes during pregnancy or deliver a child who weighed 9 pounds or more? ☐ yes ☐ no
11. Do you suffer from an autoimmune disease? ☐ yes ☐ no

Blood Type B–Specific Factors

The following factors are known to specifically influence Blood Type B's risk for obesity, insulin resistance, and diabetes. Answer yes or no to each question.

1. Do you consume a high-carbohydrate, low-protein diet? ☐ yes ☐ no
2. Do you have a history of following very low-calorie "starvation" diets? ☐ yes ☐ no
3. Are you experiencing high stress levels? ☐ yes ☐ no
4. Do you experience hypoglycemia? ☐ yes ☐ no
5. Do you lead a sedentary lifestyle that includes little aerobic exercise? ☐ yes ☐ no
6. Do you eat wheat every day? ☐ yes ☐ no
7. Do you often skip meals? ☐ yes ☐ no
8. Do you regularly consume refined sugars? ☐ yes ☐ no
9. Is your diet low in fiber (less than 3–4 servings per day)? ☐ yes ☐ no

Scoring: Add the number of "yes" responses in each list. Your score is based on the total:

12–20: High Risk You are almost certainly heading toward type 2 diabetes (if you don't already have it). You need to act now to address the factors you can control. Review the items marked "yes." Some, such as your age, ethnicity, and family history, are beyond your control. However, your high score indicates that there are major areas that you can change.

8–11: Moderate Risk If you make some changes now, you can still prevent diabetes. Review the items marked "yes," paying special attention to those related to diet, exercise, and lifestyle, to determine the actions you must take.

0–7: Low Risk Your risk is not severe. Keep it that way by following the Blood Type B Diet and lifestyle plan.

Blood Type AB Quiz
Are You Diabetes-Prone?

General Factors

The following factors are known to contribute to an individual's overall diabetes risk. Answer yes or no to each question.

1. Does a parent or sibling of yours have diabetes? ☐ yes ☐ no
2. Is your racial or ethnic background African-American, Hispanic, or Native American? ☐ yes ☐ no
3. Are you more than 20% overweight? ☐ yes ☐ no
4. Do you have high blood pressure? ☐ yes ☐ no
5. Do you have high cholesterol (overall above 200 and HDL under 45 mg/dL for men and 55 mg/dL for women)? ☐ yes ☐ no
6. Do you have a triglyceride level over 150 mg/dL? ☐ yes ☐ no

7. Are you 50 years old or older?   ☐ yes ☐ no
8. Do you have a history of heavy alcohol use?   ☐ yes ☐ no
9. Do you smoke?   ☐ yes ☐ no
10. (Women) Did you have gestational diabetes
    during pregnancy or deliver a child who
    weighed 9 pounds or more?   ☐ yes ☐ no
11. Do you suffer from an autoimmune disease?   ☐ yes ☐ no

Blood Type AB–Specific Factors

The following factors are known to specifically influence Blood Type AB's risk for obesity, insulin resistance, and diabetes. Answer yes or no to each question.

1. Do you consume a high-protein, high-fat diet?   ☐ yes ☐ no
2. Do you have a history of following very
    low-calorie "starvation" diets?   ☐ yes ☐ no
3. Do you often skip meals?   ☐ yes ☐ no
4. Do you often experience hypoglycemia?   ☐ yes ☐ no
5. Do you avoid exercise, even stretching
    or yoga?   ☐ yes ☐ no
6. Do you eat meat every day?   ☐ yes ☐ no
7. Do you regularly consume refined sugars?   ☐ yes ☐ no
8. Is your diet low in fiber (less than 3–4 servings
    per day)?   ☐ yes ☐ no
9. Do you need stimulants (coffee, chocolate,
    cigarettes, etc.) to keep you going?   ☐ yes ☐ no

Scoring: Add the number of "yes" responses in each list. Your score is based on the total:

12–20: High Risk You are almost certainly heading toward type 2 diabetes (if you don't already have it). You need to act now to address the factors you can control. Review the items marked "yes." Some, such as your age, ethnicity, and family history, are beyond your control. However, your high score indicates that there are major areas that you can change.

8–11: Moderate Risk If you make some changes now, you can still prevent diabetes. Review the items marked "yes," paying special attention to those related to diet, exercise, and lifestyle, to determine the actions you must take.

0–7: Low Risk Your risk is not severe. Keep it that way by following the Blood Type AB Diet and lifestyle plan.

Blood Type and Diabetes: A Basic Primer

Blood Type
and Diabetes:
A Basic Primer

The
Dynamics
of Diabetes

THE BLOOD TYPE DIET MAY OFFER THE MOST EFFECTIVE approach yet in controlling the epidemic of diabetes. Although the numbers of those afflicted have been on the rise in recent years, 90 percent of all diabetes is preventable by eating the right diet and exercising appropriately. Furthermore, new research by the National Institutes of Health shows that even people who have an exceptionally high genetic propensity to develop diabetes can reduce their risk by almost 60 percent through diet and lifestyle adjustments. Imagine that. We have the power to virtually eliminate the damaging effects of diabetes by making simple changes in the way we eat and live.

The progression to full-fledged diabetes usually occurs over time, so the Blood Type Diet can have a dramatic preventive influence. If you are reading this book, you may already have diabetes, but it is more likely that you are pre-diabetic and want to stop the progression of the disease in its tracks. In a pre-diabetic stage, you're probably overweight, and you may experience the symptoms of blood sugar irregularity.

A blood test may show higher than normal levels of blood glucose—a sign of impending or prolonged hyperglycemia. If you remain in this state of prolonged hyperglycemia, diabetes is inevitable.

That's where the Blood Type Diet comes in. Extensive research and clinical testing has shown conclusively that when you adhere to a diet that maximizes your utilization of food, you can reverse the slide into full-fledged diabetes. The Blood Type Diet is the only individualized approach to diabetes prevention and management currently available. Unlike other diet plans, which propose one plan to fit everyone, the Blood Type Diet addresses the critical genetic differences, which influence the way your body metabolizes food.

Diabetes: A Problem with Food

DIABETES IS A DISEASE that impairs your body's ability to use food efficiently. The hormone insulin, which is produced in the pancreas, helps your body change food into energy. Diabetes occurs when one of two conditions exists: either your pancreas fails to make insulin, or your body cannot properly use the insulin it does make.

To understand why insulin is important, it helps to know more about how food is used for energy. Your body is made up of millions of cells. To make energy, these cells need food in a very simple form. Much of the food you eat is broken down into a simple sugar called glucose. Glucose provides the energy you need for daily activities.

When you eat, your pancreas releases insulin into the bloodstream, which helps to break down and absorb glucose, fatty acids, and amino acids. If your pancreas does not produce insulin, or if your body can't properly employ it, the foods you eat can't be metabolized. When you produce insulin but do not react to it, the resulting condition is called insulin resistance. This is common in many obese individuals as their bodies begin to age. You need to produce more and more insulin to less effect. Eventually, excess glucose collects in the blood, instead of being used for energy or stored as fat. That's why diabetics have high blood sugar. If there is too much glucose in your blood, it can't be processed by the kidneys and is excreted in your urine. The proper term for the disease, diabetes mellitus, means literally "flowing with honey," referring to the amount of sugar excreted in the urine. In days gone by, before glucose tests and urine strips, intrepid physicians would often taste the patient's urine for a characteristic sweetish taste as a way to diagnose diabetes. Talk about job dedication!

Diabetes is actually two different diseases. Type 1 diabetes is a failure to produce insulin. Type 2 diabetes is a failure to utilize insulin. Gestational diabetes is often referred to as a third form, but it is actually linked to type 2 diabetes. Gestational diabetes is a temporary condition of insulin resistance that usually occurs halfway through a pregnancy as a result of excessive hormone production, or the inability of the pancreas to make the additional insulin that is needed. Gestational diabetes usually goes away after pregnancy, but women who have had gestational diabetes are at an increased risk for later developing type 2 diabetes.

Most of the preventative focus is on type 2 diabetes, which accounts for the majority of cases and which can be avoided with the right diet. It is not so clear how type 1 diabetes can be prevented. However, both forms of diabetes can be more easily managed if you adhere to the diet that is right for your blood type.

Type 1 Diabetes: An Immune Disorder

TYPE 1 DIABETES, formerly known as juvenile or insulin-dependent diabetes, occurs when the pancreas is unable to produce insulin. It usually begins in childhood or young adulthood and lasts throughout a diabetic's life. Type 1 accounts for about 10 percent of all diabetes cases.

Type 1 diabetes is caused by destruction of the beta cells in the pancreas that are responsible for the secretion of insulin. It is believed to be, at least initially, an autoimmune disease triggered by a toxin or virus. This "event" prompts the body's immune system to attack the pancreas. The beta cells of the pancreas are so damaged in the attack that they are no longer able to produce insulin.

Initial signs of type 1 diabetes include extreme thirst and hunger, unexplained weight loss, frequent copious urination, blurred vision, fatigue, and chronic infections. In a crisis situation, the onset of type 1 diabetes may cause convulsions, confusion, slurred speech, fruity-smelling breath, and unconsciousness.

Type 1 diabetes can only be controlled by the use of injected insulin and daily food monitoring. It is not curable, but careful management allows diabetics to live normal lives.

Type 2 Diabetes: A Metabolic Disorder

UNLIKE PEOPLE WITH type 1 diabetes, people with type 2 diabetes produce insulin. However, the insulin they produce either is not enough or doesn't work properly in the body. When there isn't enough insulin, or the insulin is not used as it should be, glucose can't get into the body's cells.

Type 2 diabetes is most often seen in overweight men and women over forty years of age. Until recently, type 2 diabetes was known as "adult-onset diabetes," because it was unheard of in children. But in the past decade, researchers have seen an alarming rise in the numbers of overweight and obese children and teenagers who have the disease. (This seismic shift is also the reason type 1 diabetes is no longer called "juvenile" diabetes.)

Type 2 diabetes can be a gateway to several other life-threatening conditions. Chief among them is the heightened risk of developing coronary artery disease (CAD). CAD is the leading cause of death among people with diabetes. When you have uncontrolled high blood sugar from diabetes, it can do systemic damage to your body. Over the years, it can lead to heart attacks and strokes at an early age, blindness, foot and leg amputations, and kidney failure.

Pre-Diabetes: The Warning Signs

ALTHOUGH PEOPLE with type 1 diabetes almost always suspect they are ill, type 2 diabetes can develop gradually over a period of months or years, and you might not realize there's anything seriously wrong until it's well advanced. Typical symptoms include increased thirst and hunger, frequent urination, unexplained weight loss, blurred vision, and recurrent urinary tract infections.

Often, doctors are able to detect the likelihood of type 2 diabetes before the condition actually occurs. You'll be diagnosed with pre-diabetes when your blood glucose levels are higher than normal but not high enough for a diagnosis of type 2 diabetes. This condition is called *hyperglycemia.* Low blood sugar, or *hypoglycemia,* is not a symptom of pre-diabetes. This is a subject of some confusion among my patients, because the term hypoglycemia has been widely and casually used to refer to everything from hunger headaches to post-meal sleepiness. In fact, diabetes-related hypoglycemia usually occurs as a side effect of medications that lower blood sugar. If medications are overprescribed, or you fail to monitor your blood sugar, skip meals, or eat the wrong foods, your blood sugar levels can drop too low to provide energy for your body's needs. The clinical diagnosis of pre-diabetes is related to high blood sugar.

How do you know if you should be tested for pre-diabetes? There are clear signals:

Are You Overweight?

Obesity is the number one sign that you may be pre-diabetic. Obesity is *always* accompanied by insulin resistance, which leads to diabetes. When it comes to body fat and insulin resistance, the easiest way to think of this problem is in terms of a sliding scale: more body fat = more insulin resistance.

According to a 2003 report by the Centers for Disease Control, the obesity and diabetes epidemics have continued to escalate. Currently, more than 44 million Americans are considered obese, an increase of 74 percent since 1991. During the same time frame, diabetes increased by 61 percent, reflecting the strong correlation between the two.

Obesity upsets the regulation of energy metabolism in two ways: It produces leptin resistance and it promotes insulin resistance. Leptin (not to be confused with "lectin," an important concept we will get to later) is a hormone associated with the obesity gene and has been receiving a lot of research attention in recent years. Leptin acts on the hypothalamus to regulate the extent of body fat, the ability to burn fat for energy, and satiety (the feeling of having eaten enough).

When you're overweight, your leptin levels increase, but its action is stifled. In obesity, leptin levels increase in concert with insulin levels, leading some researchers to believe that leptin resistance is the precursor to insulin resistance. Leptin is also associated with the stress hormone cortisol. As a general rule, when you are overweight you will have chronically

> **MEASURE YOUR HIP-WAIST RATIO**
> Excess weight is most unhealthy—and most conducive to metabolic problems—when it is centered in your abdomen, as opposed to your hips and thighs. Here's a quick test to learn about your fat distribution: Stand straight in front of a full-length mirror. Using a tape measure, measure the distance around the smallest part of your waist. Now measure the distance around the largest part of your buttocks. Divide your waist measurement by your hip measurement. A healthy ratio for women is .70 to .75. A healthy ratio for men is .80 to .90.

elevated levels of cortisol. Fat tissue accelerates the production of cortisol, and high levels of cortisol promote weight gain. It's a vicious cycle. Cortisol differs from other steroid hormones, such as sex hormones, in that it is classified as a glucocorticoid. That means its primary action involves increasing blood sugar levels at the expense of muscle tissue. While this is the desired effect in a fight-or-flight situation, on a chronic basis it will lead to insulin resistance and an alteration in body composition from muscle to fat. In addition, research shows that high cortisol tends to increase your appetite, because of an association with leptin. Research suggests that cortisol is the primary factor that prevents leptin from suppressing appetite, increasing metabolism, and decreasing body fat.

Do You Have Too Much Fat in the Abdominal Area?

Even normal-weight individuals can be pre-diabetic when they have excess fat in the wrong places. Studies show that a preponderance of fat in the gut is related to a heightened diabetes risk among normal-weight individuals. These people are considered "metabolically obese" despite their weight.

Do You Have a Sluggish Metabolism?

Your Basal Metabolic Rate (BMR) is the number of calories that you would burn during the course of a day while at rest. As a general rule, BMR tends to decline with age, due mostly to loss of muscle mass. A high ratio of active tissue mass to body fat translates into a more aggressive antifat metabolism, because more muscle tissue increases the rate and amount of fat you use for fuel while you are at rest. Metabolically active tissue is defined as muscle tissue and organ tissues—such as liver, brain, and heart—which actively burn fuel. Some of the advantages of an increased active tissue mass include more strength, increased metabolic rate, increased aerobic capacity, improved cardiovascular health, better utilization of insulin, and healthier cholesterol counts.

Maintaining a high percentage of active tissue is particularly important when you are trying to lose weight. With diets that severely restrict calories, you may lose weight but also lose muscle tissue. Since these diets do nothing to increase active tissue mass, your metabolic rate remains unchanged or declines, leaving you predisposed to regain the weight you lost (or perhaps more) as soon as you resume normal eating.

Are You Bloated, Especially After Meals?

In a healthy state, your cells are well hydrated. Intracellular water keeps your metabolism operating efficiently. However, extracellular water—which is fluid buildup outside your cells—is unhealthy. This condition, known as edema, is the result of obesity, eating the wrong foods, skipping meals, a sedentary lifestyle, and "yo-yo" dieting.

EACH OF THESE factors is a sign that your body is not utilizing food properly. Most prediabetics will have one or more of these symptoms. If you are over

TEST FOR EXTRACELLULAR WATER—EDEMA

Push your finger firmly down on your shin bone and hold it for five seconds. If you push against muscle or fat, the skin will bounce back up. If there is water between the cells, it will be displaced laterally, and the dimple won't fill in immediately. The longer the indentation remains, the more water is present, meaning you're holding excess weight as water.

forty, your risk of developing full-fledged diabetes from these conditions is even greater.

The Complications of Diabetes

DIABETES BECOMES DEADLY because of its sweeping effects on other body systems. In recent years, medical researchers have given increasing attention to a condition they refer to as Metabolic Syndrome (formerly called Syndrome X). Metabolic Syndrome, which affects about 47 million Americans, is a clustering of problems that together form a dangerous and potentially deadly state. These conditions include insulin resistance, high blood sugar, elevated triglycerides, high LDL (low-density lipoproteins) cholesterol, low HDL (high-density lipoproteins) cholesterol, high blood pressure, and obesity (especially abdominal fat). Metabolic Syndrome is the gateway to heart disease. Most diabetics have at least one or two additional conditions and need to monitor them to reduce the risk of heart disease.

Metabolic Syndrome Involves at Least Three of the Following:

- Waist more than 40 inches around in men or 35 inches in women
- Triglyceride levels of 150 or greater
- HDL, or "good" cholesterol, less than 40 in men or less than 50 in women
- Blood pressure of 130/85 or more
- Fasting blood sugar of 100 or more

Normal Blood Pressure	Less than 119/79
Pre-Hypertension	120/80 to 139/89
Mild Hypertension	140/90 to 159/99
Moderate Hypertension	160/100 to 179/109
Severe Hypertension	180/110 and above

Diabetics have been shown to have higher mean blood pressure. In African-American diabetics, hypertension is especially widespread, affecting between 63 and 70 percent of diabetics.

People with diabetes often have high cholesterol and/or high triglycerides. Your body uses cholesterol to build cell walls and to produce certain vitamins and hormones. Your body uses triglycerides as stored fat. Stored fat keeps you warm, protects your body's organs, and gives you energy reserves. When lipids are out of control, they collect and harden into arterial plaque, which blocks the flow of blood to the heart.

Heart disease is the leading cause of death among diabetics and is closely linked with other factors, such as high cholesterol, high blood pressure, and high triglycerides. It was once believed that high risk of heart disease mostly occurred among older people with type 2 diabetes. However, new research shows that one out of ten young people with type 1 diabetes show early signs of heart disease. Diabetics—both type 1 and type 2—are two to four times as likely to suffer heart attacks as the general population.

Diabetes can also cause nerve damage, which leads to impaired blood flow and numbness in the legs and feet. Long-term or older diabetics tend to have severe circulation problems due to impaired blood flow through small arteries. This increases their susceptibility to foot injuries, which are slow to heal and in danger of becoming infected. Diabetes is the direct cause of some 40,000 leg and foot amputations a year in older men and women. A new study by the National Center for Chronic Disease Prevention and Health Promotion at the Centers for Disease Control shows that 67 percent of all amputees are diabetics.

> **THE HEALTHIEST**
> **BLOOD FAT LEVELS ARE**
> Total cholesterol under 200 mg/dL
> LDL cholesterol under 130 mg/dL
> HDL cholesterol over 35 mg/dL
> Triglycerides under 200 mg/dL

Over time, high blood sugar levels can damage the kidneys, which act as filters to clean the blood of waste products and extra fluid. When kidneys are damaged, this purifying job is impaired and waste products build up in the blood. People who have kidney failure must have dialysis treatment or receive a kidney transplant. Kidney failure is often a fatal complication for elderly patients with severe diabetes.

High blood sugar can eventually damage the blood vessels that feed the retina of the eye. In early stages, the blood vessels may begin to leak fluid, and there may be swelling and blurred vision. In advanced stages, abnormal blood vessels grow on the retina and block vision.

How Is Diabetes Diagnosed?

THE STANDARD SCREENING METHOD for diabetes is the fasting blood glucose test, which measures the amount of glucose in your blood after you've abstained from food for a period of ten to twelve hours. Your blood is taken and sent to a lab for analysis. Normal fasting blood glucose is between 70 and 100 milligrams per deciliter (mg/dL). The standard diagnosis of diabetes is made when two separate blood tests show that your fasting blood glucose level is greater than or equal to 126 mg/dL.

While the fasting plasma glucose test is the most accurate, a casual plasma glucose test can be taken without abstaining from food. With this test, a glucose level greater than 200 mg/dL may indicate diabetes, especially if the test is repeated at a later time and shows similar results.

Some people have a normal fasting blood glucose reading, but their blood glucose rapidly rises as they eat. These people may have glucose intolerance, determined through the use of the glucose tolerance test. A glucose tolerance test takes several hours. Subjects are given a sugary liquid to swallow, which temporarily produces high blood sugar. Then, blood samples are taken at intervals of 30 minutes, one hour, two hours, and three hours, and the glucose level is measured in each sample. This tells how quickly the body is able to bring the blood sugar level back down to normal.

The Blood Type– Diabetes Connection

WHAT DOES YOUR BLOOD TYPE HAVE TO DO WITH YOUR risk for diabetes? Quite a bit, as it turns out. Your blood type is a key modulator of your digestive system, your metabolic activity, and your immunity. Think of it as your physiological balancing factor.

Each blood type is determined by a chemical marker called an antigen. Most people also carry antibodies against the antigens of the other blood types. These blood type antibodies are not there to complicate transfusions, but rather to protect your body against foreign substances such as bacteria, viruses, parasites, and some foods, which actually resemble foreign blood type antigens. When your immune system encounters one of these substances that resembles a blood type opposed to yours, it creates antibodies against it. This antibody reaction occurs through a process of agglutination. That is, the antibody you create will attach to the foreign substance and dispose of it.

Scientists have also learned that many foods contain proteins called lectins, which can agglutinate the cells of certain blood types but not others—meaning that a food may be harmful to the cells of one blood type, but beneficial to the cells of another. This discovery of the link between blood type and diet has significant implications for the prevention and management of diabetes.

Different Blood Types, Different Pathways

THERE ARE IMPORTANT differences among the blood types in the risk factors for diabetes, as well as in the pathways to the disease.

Blood Types A and AB

From a purely statistical standpoint, Blood Type A and to a slightly lesser degree Blood Type AB are at higher risk than the other blood types for both type 1 and type 2 diabetes. This ABO-mediated susceptibility is especially strong in males. This association has been confirmed in several large independent studies, examining and tracking literally thousands of people.

An important reason why type 1 diabetes is more prevalent in Blood Type A individuals is the potential for maternal-child blood type incompatibility. A recent study of almost 400 juvenile diabetics showed that an amazing 90 percent are parents whose blood types were incompatible with the child's. Since any mother-fetus "hostility"—occurring when a fetus carries a blood type to which the mother's immune system is reactive—would compromise the proper formation of tissue and organs, it is likely that the mother's immune system triggers the destruction of the insulin-producing cells of the pancreas while the infant is still in utero. The consequences of maternal-fetal incompatibility are most severe when the mother is Blood Type O and the child is Blood Type A.

Type 2 diabetes has a different set of risk factors. Blood Type A, and to a lesser extent Blood Type AB, genetically favors a diet that is low in animal protein and high in complex carbohydrates and high-quality vegetable protein, such as soy. These blood types lack the digestive enzymes to properly metabolize a high-fat, high-protein diet. When Blood Types A and AB overconsume meat, it increases their overall cholesterol and their LDL cholesterol. In combination with their general tendency to have blood that clots more readily, these factors give Blood Type A and AB diabetics a greater risk of developing cardiovascular and arterial complications due to diabetes.

Our strategies for Blood Types A and AB focus primarily on preventing and managing type 2 diabetes. Can you do anything to reduce the effects of maternal-fetal incompatibility that may lead to type 1 diabetes? Following your diet prior to pregnancy is a good start. (For more information about maternal-fetal blood type compatibility, consult my book *Eat Right 4 Your Baby: The Individualized Guide to Fertility and Maximum Health During Pregnancy, Nursing, and Your Baby's First Year.*)

Blood Types O and B

Carbohydrate intolerance is the main pathway to diabetes for Blood Types O and B. In this respect, they are the opposite of Blood Types A and AB. Since they are unable to fully digest many carbohydrate foods (particularly grains and beans), these foods are converted to fat.

The typical Blood Type O or B patient I treat who has diabetes or a pre-diabetic condition is overweight and has high triglycerides and blood pressure. Obesity itself is a major sign of insulin resistance. Diabetes is believed to be the leading cause of hypertriglyceridemia (chronic high triglycerides), and this is particularly true for Blood Types O and B. In other words, insulin resistance, caused by carbohydrate intolerance, leads to high triglycerides.

A classic sign of insulin resistance in Blood Types O and B is the "apple-shaped figure," characterized by a broad girth at the mid-section. "Pear-shaped" individuals, with fat located in the hips and thighs, do not have the same health risks. Fat cells located in the abdomen release fat into the blood more easily than fat cells found elsewhere. The release of fat from the abdomen begins within three to four hours after a meal is consumed, compared to many more hours for other fat cells. This early release shows up as higher triglycerides and free fatty acid levels. Free fatty acids themselves cause insulin resistance, and elevated triglycerides usually coincide with low HDL cholesterol. The strategies for Blood Types O and B will focus on fighting type 2 diabetes, primarily by preventing carbohydrate intolerance.

Secretors and Non-Secretors

PEOPLE WHO DO NOT secrete blood type antigens (about 20 percent of the population) are at a greater risk of developing diabetes, especially type 2 diabetes. They are also more likely to develop complications when they do suffer from diabetes. Non-diabetics with glucose intolerance are also significantly more likely to be non-secretors.

Many Blood Type O and Blood Type B non-secretors have insulin resistance syndrome, which can cause impairment of triglyceride conversion, resulting in a lowered metabolic rate. Low metabolism also promotes the storage of excess fluid as extracellular water, leading to edema.

For more information about the implications of your secretor status, refer to the *Eat Right 4 Your Type Complete Blood Type Encyclopedia*.

The Diabetes-Stress Factor

BLOOD TYPE A and to some extent Blood Type B have an additional risk factor for diabetes: naturally elevated levels of the stress hormone cortisol. For these blood types, being in a condition of stress can create metabolic havoc. That's because stress hormones promote insulin resistance and hormonal imbalance. They also signal the body to metabolize muscle tissue. Obesity itself leads to cortisol resistance; it becomes a dangerously vicious cycle. High cortisol, as we discussed earlier, is also associated with leptin. High cortisol = lowered sensitivity to leptin = increased appetite.

A deeper discussion of blood type and stress is available in the book *Live Right 4 Your Type: The Individualized Prescription for Maximizing Health, Metabolism, and Vitality in Every Stage of Your Life.*

The Lectin Trigger

INSULIN RESISTANCE is often triggered by the overconsumption of lectin-containing foods that react unfavorably with your blood type. Lectins—abundant and diverse proteins found in foods—have agglutinating properties that affect your blood. Lectins are a powerful way for organisms in nature to attach themselves to other organisms in nature. They are used by microbes in much the same way our own immune systems use them. For example, cells in the liver's bile ducts have lectins on their surfaces to help them snatch up bacteria and parasites.

So, too, with the lectins in food. Simply put, when you eat a food containing protein lectins that are reactive with your blood type antigen, the lectins passing through the gut wall enter the circulation, and target an organ or organ system (kidneys, liver, thyroid, etc.). They begin to agglutinate blood cells in that area.

Some lectins—particularly those found in many common grains—can wreak havoc on the body's fat cells by binding to their insulin receptors. Once they bind to the receptors, they signal fat cells to stop burning fat and to store extra calories as fat. Consuming large amounts of insulin-mimicking lectins that are wrong for your blood type will promote insulin resistance.

The Blood Type Diet offers an individualized way to attack insulin resistance, pre-diabetes, and diabetes. In the following pages, you will learn how you can use blood type–specific guidelines as a key component of your diabetes-fighting effort.

THREE

Fighting Diabetes with Conventional and Blood Type Therapies

THE BLOOD TYPE DIET IS THE CENTERPIECE OF AN ANTIdiabetes strategy, whether your goal is preventing the disease or managing it. Your individualized blood type plan will help you attain metabolic balance and maximize the efficient use of the food you eat. Although there is no cure for diabetes, I have found that the Blood Type Diet enables many of my patients to manage the disease so well that they are able to minimize or even avoid taking medications for type 2 diabetes. And although there is currently no effective natural treatment alternative for injectable insulin replacement for type 1 diabetics, the diet and naturopathic supplement program I have devised has helped my patients avoid many of the complications stemming from lifelong diabetes, such as cataracts, neuropathy, and cardiovascular problems.

If you are currently under medical supervision and are taking medications or injectable insulin, the Blood Type Diet and lifestyle guidelines specified for your blood type can provide an excellent support system. Most of my patients use the best conventional medicine has to offer, along with the added benefits of a diet that is genetically suited to their needs.

Conventional Treatment Protocols

IN CONVENTIONAL MEDICINE, diabetes is usually treated in one of two ways—with injected insulin or with oral medications. Injected insulin is required for type 1 diabetes and for the most severe cases of type 2 diabetes. Most type 2 diabetics are prescribed one or more oral medications. Diabetes medications are grouped into categories based on medication type. There are several categories of oral diabetes medicine:

- Sulfonylureas include: first-generation medicine (Dymelor, Diabinese, Orinase, Tolinase) and second-generation medicine (Glucotrol, Glucotrol XL, DiaBeta, Micronase, Glynase PresTab, and Amaryl). These drugs lower blood glucose by stimulating the pancreas to release more insulin.
- Biguanides include Glucophage, Glucophage XR, and metformin. These drugs improve insulin's ability to move glucose into cells, especially in the liver.
- Sulfonylureas and biguanide combination, such as Glucovance. This drug stimulates the pancreas to release more insulin, improves insulin's action in the body, and lowers the amount of glucose released by the liver.
- Thiazolidinediones Actos and Avandia. These drugs improve insulin's effectiveness (decreasing insulin resistance) and lower the amount of glucose produced by the liver. (According to recent research, this class of drugs may have potentially dangerous side effects.)

- Alpha-glucosidase inhibitors, including Precose and Glyset. These drugs block enzymes that help digest starches, slowing the rise in blood glucose. These drugs may cause diarrhea or gas.

So far, only one drug, Glucophage, has been approved to treat the effects of diabetes in kids.

Fighting Diabetes with the Blood Type Diet

THE BLOOD TYPE DIET is designed to work in a complementary fashion with any of these medications. If you are being treated for diabetes, you already know that the right diet and exercise regimen goes hand in hand with your medications. I'd recommend that before you begin this program, you sit down with your doctor and dietitian and make sure you're all on the same page. Devise a schedule for checking your progress on the Blood Type Diet. Over time, your medications may have to be adjusted. A note of caution: Never reduce or discontinue a medication without consulting your physician.

The Blood Type Diet will help you lose weight and gain active tissue mass by including only the most efficiently digested and metabolized foods for your blood type. For many diabetics and pre-diabetics, weight loss is the most important initial goal they can set. In most cases, weight loss will produce a simultaneous reduction in HDL cholesterol and triglyceride levels. Most people who start the Blood Type Diet find that they immediately begin to lose weight.

Whether you're diabetic or pre-diabetic, the Blood Type Diet will almost certainly improve the way you feel. As the seesaw effects of high to low blood sugar resolve into a controlled norm, you'll have more energy, be less moody, and be able to enjoy—perhaps for the first time in years—that delightful state of normal.

Are you ready to start? Find your blood type section, and we'll get you on the right diet for your type to fight diabetes.

PART II

Individualized Blood Type Plans

FOUR

Blood Type

O

THE PATHWAY TO DIABETES FOR BLOOD TYPE O INVOLVES carbohydrate intolerance, leading to insulin resistance; a susceptibility to thyroid regulation problems that upset your metabolic balance; and high triglycerides. Your genetic heritage is grounded in the legacy of the feast-and-famine existence of your hunter ancestors. Your metabolic health is dependent on maintaining high active tissue mass and low body fat.

For Blood Type O, insulin resistance is often the result of consuming dietary lectins that have insulinlike effects on their fat cell receptors. Unlike insulin, which "docks" only temporarily on fat cell receptors, these lectins bind persistently to the receptor, continually signaling fat cells to stop burning fat and to store extra calories as fat. In effect, eating these lectins results in your body scavenging any extra sugars/carbohydrates and converting them to unwanted fat. Blood Type O is particularly vulnerable to the insulin-mimicking lectins in grains and beans. When your diet favors these foods over the protein-rich foods

Blood Type O Weight Profile

Weight Gain		Weight Loss	
FOOD	MECHANISM	FOOD	MECHANISM
Wheat	Insulin resistance	Red meat	Aids efficient metabolism, builds muscle
Corn	Insulin resistance	Walnuts	Improve insulin metabolism
Dairy	Poorly digested	Broccoli, kale, spinach	Aid efficient metabolism
Kidney and navy beans, lentils	Insulin resistance, impairs calorie utilization	Seaweeds, seafoods, sea salt	Increase thyroid hormone production
Cabbage, Brussels sprouts, cauliflower	Inhibit thyroid hormone	Plum, pineapple	Improve insulin metabolism

that are well metabolized by your blood type, you will gain weight and have trouble metabolizing sugars. Insulin resistance syndrome also impairs triglyceride conversion and promotes the storage of excess fluid, causing edema.

Insulin-resistant Blood Type Os have an added problem with thyroid regulation. You tend to have naturally low levels of thyroid hormone, making you susceptible to hypothyroidism. Insulin resistance also slows thyroid activity, worsening your condition.

Blood Type O: The Foods

THE BLOOD TYPE O Diabetes Diet is specifically adapted for the prevention and management of diabetes. A new category, **Super Beneficial,** highlights powerful disease-fighting foods for Blood Type O. The **Neutral** category has also been adjusted to de-emphasize foods that can cause problems for diabetics. Foods designated **Neutral: Allowed Infrequently** should be minimized or avoided entirely.

Food Values

SUPER BENEFICIAL	Foods that are known to have specific disease-fighting qualities for your blood type.
BENEFICIAL	Foods with components that enhance the metabolic, immune, or structural health of your blood type.
NEUTRAL: Allowed Frequently	Foods that normally have no direct blood type effect but supply a variety of nutrients necessary for a healthful diet.
NEUTRAL: Allowed Infrequently	Foods that normally have no blood type effect but may impede your progress when consumed regularly.
AVOID	Foods with components that are harmful to your blood type.

Your secretor status can influence your ability to fully digest and metabolize certain foods, so various adjustments in the values are made for non-secretors. If you do not know your secretor type, the odds are that you can safely use the "secretor" values, since the majority of the population (80 percent) are secretors. However, I urge you to get tested, since the variations are important for non-secretors who want to maximize the effectiveness of the Blood Type Diet.

The food charts are divided into three sections. The top of the chart suggests the average portion size and quantity per week or day, according to secretor status. These recommendations do *not* apply to the category **Neutral: Allowed Infrequently;** those foods should be consumed sparingly (0–2 times per month). The charts also indicate differences in frequency for some foods, based on ethnic heritage. It has been my experience that this factor has an impact on the individual's ability to fully digest certain foods. For the purposes of blood type food choices, persons of Hispanic heritage should follow the recommendations for Caucasians, and North American Native peoples should follow the recommendations for Asians.

The middle section of the chart suggests food values. The bottom section lists variants based on secretor status.

For your convenience, we have included a number of product names, such as ketchup, Worcestershire sauce, and Ezekiel bread. However, bear in mind that commercial formulations vary among brands and regions. Even though a product may be listed as okay for you, always check its ingredients; do not use products that contain **Avoid** ingredients for your blood type. Of course, you may choose to make your own version of commercial products, such as bread and mayonnaise, using ingredients that suit your blood type. There are hundreds of delicious recipes for every blood type available on our Web site (www.dadamo.com) and in the book *Cook Right 4 Your Type: The Practical Kitchen Companion to* Eat Right 4 Your Type.

Meat/Poultry

Protein is critical for Blood Type O. Inadequate protein intake can seriously interfere with your ability to metabolize fats, leading to insulin resistance and diabetes. For Blood Type O, high-quality protein is one of the best preventative measures to take against obesity. Protein increases active tissue mass, which increases your basal metabolic rate, enabling excess fat to be burned off more quickly. Choose only the best-quality (preferably grass-fed), chemical-, antibiotic-, and pesticide-free, low-fat meats and poultry.

BLOOD TYPE O: MEAT/POULTRY			
Portion: 4–6 oz (men); 2–5 oz (women and children)			
	African	Caucasian	Asian
Secretor	6–9	6–9	6–9
Non-Secretor	7–12	7–12	7–11
		Times per week	

SUPER BENEFICIAL	BENEFICIAL	NEUTRAL: Allowed Frequently	NEUTRAL: Allowed Infrequently	AVOID
Beef	Heart	Chicken		All com-
Buffalo	(calf)	Cornish		mercially
Lamb	Sweet-	hen		processed
Liver (calf)	breads	Duck		meats
Mutton	Venison	Goat		Bacon/Ham/
Veal		Goose		Pork
		Grouse		Quail
		Guinea		Turtle
		hen		
		Horse		
		Ostrich		
		Partridge		
		Pheasant		
		Rabbit		
		Squab		
		Squirrel		
		Turkey		

Special Variants: *Non-Secretor* BENEFICIAL: ostrich, partridge; NEUTRAL (Allowed Frequently): lamb, liver (calf), quail, turtle.

Fish/Seafood

Fish and other seafoods represent a secondary source of high-quality protein for Blood Type O. In particular, richly oiled cold-water fish, containing beneficial oils, can improve your metabolism, blood flow, and thyroid function.

BLOOD TYPE O: FISH/SEAFOOD			
Portion: 4–6 oz (men); 2–5 oz (women and children)			
	African	Caucasian	Asian
Secretor	2–4	3–5	2–5
Non-Secretor	2–5	4–5	4–5
		Times per week	

SUPER BENEFICIAL	BENEFICIAL	NEUTRAL: Allowed Frequently	NEUTRAL: Allowed Infrequently	AVOID
Cod	Bass (all)	Anchovy	Eel	Abalone
Halibut	Perch (all)	Beluga	Flounder	Barracuda
Red snapper	Pike	Bluefish	Gray sole	Catfish
Trout (rainbow)	Shad	Bullhead	Grouper	Conch
	Sole (except gray)	Butterfish	Whitefish	Frog
	Sturgeon	Carp		Herring (pickled/ smoked)
	Swordfish	Caviar (sturgeon)		Muskel-lunge
	Tilefish	Chub		Octopus
	Yellowtail	Clam		Pollock
		Crab		Salmon (smoked)
		Croaker		Squid (calamari)
		Cusk		
		Drum		
		Haddock		
		Hake		
		Halfmoon fish		
		Harvest fish		
		Herring (fresh)		
		Lobster		
		Mackerel		
		Mahi-mahi		
		Monkfish		
		Mullet		
		Mussel		
		Opaleye		
		Orange roughy		
		Oyster		
		Parrot fish		

SUPER BENEFICIAL	BENEFICIAL	NEUTRAL: Allowed Frequently	NEUTRAL: Allowed Infrequently	AVOID
		Pickerel		
		Pompano		
		Porgy		
		Rosefish		
		Sailfish		
		Salmon		
		Salmon roe		
		Sardine		
		Scallop		
		Scrod		
		Shark		
		Shrimp		
		Smelt		
		Snail (*Helix pomatia/* escargot)		
		Sucker		
		Sunfish		
		Tilapia		
		Trout (brook, sea)		
		Tuna		
		Weakfish		
		Whiting		

Special Variants: *Non-Secretor* BENEFICIAL: hake, herring (fresh), mackerel, sardine; NEUTRAL (Allowed Frequently): bass, catfish, halibut, red snapper, salmon roe; AVOID: anchovy, crab, mussel.

Dairy/Eggs

Most dairy foods should be avoided by Blood Type O. They are poorly digested, contributing to weight gain, increased inflammation, and fatigue. Eggs can be consumed in moderation. They are a good source of docosahexaenoic acid (DHA), and can help you build active tissue mass. Do your best to find eggs and dairy products that meet organic standards.

BLOOD TYPE O: EGGS			
Portion: 1 egg			
	African	Caucasian	Asian
Secretor	1–4	3–6	3–4
Non-Secretor	2–5	3–6	3–4
		Times per week	

BLOOD TYPE O: MILK AND YOGURT			
Portion: 4–6 oz (men); 2–5 oz (women and children)			
	African	Caucasian	Asian
Secretor	0–1	0–3	0–2
Non-Secretor	0	0–2	0–3
		Times per week	

BLOOD TYPE O: CHEESE			
Portion: 3 oz (men); 2 oz (women and children)			
	African	Caucasian	Asian
Secretor	0–1	0–2	0–1
Non-Secretor	0	0–1	0
		Times per week	

SUPER BENEFICIAL	BENEFICIAL	NEUTRAL: Allowed Frequently	NEUTRAL: Allowed Infrequently	AVOID
	Ghee (clarified butter)	Egg (chicken/ duck)	Butter Farmer cheese Feta Goat cheese Mozzarella	American cheese Blue cheese Brie Buttermilk Camembert

SUPER BENEFICIAL	BENEFICIAL	NEUTRAL: Allowed Frequently	NEUTRAL: Allowed Infrequently	AVOID
				Casein
				Cheddar
				Colby
				Cottage cheese
				Cream cheese
				Edam
				Egg (goose/ quail)
				Emmenthal
				Gouda
				Gruyère
				Half-and-half
				Ice cream
				Jarlsberg
				Kefir
				Milk (cow/ goat)
				Monterey Jack
				Muenster
				Neufchâtel
				Paneer
				Parmesan
				Provolone
				Quark
				Ricotta
				Sherbet
				Sour cream
				String cheese
				Swiss cheese

SUPER BENEFICIAL	BENEFICIAL	NEUTRAL: Allowed Frequently	NEUTRAL: Allowed Infrequently	AVOID
				Whey
				Yogurt (all)

Special Variants: *Non-Secretor* NEUTRAL (Allowed Frequently): Egg (goose/quail); AVOID: farmer cheese, feta, goat cheese, mozzarella.

Oils

Concentrate on healthy oils for Blood Type O. These are monounsaturated oils (such as olive oil) and oils rich in omega series fatty acids (such as flax oil).

BLOOD TYPE O: OILS

Portion: 1 tblsp

	African	Caucasian	Asian
Secretor	3–8	4–8	5–8
Non-Secretor	1–7	3–5	3–6
	Times per week		

SUPER BENEFICIAL	BENEFICIAL	NEUTRAL: Allowed Frequently	NEUTRAL: Allowed Infrequently	AVOID
Borage seed	Olive	Almond	Canola	Castor
Flax (lin-seed)		Black currant seed		Coconut
		Cod liver		Corn
		Sesame		Cottonseed
		Walnut		Evening primrose
				Peanut
				Safflower
				Soy
				Sunflower
				Wheat germ

Special Variants: *Non-Secretor* BENEFICIAL: almond, walnut; NEUTRAL (Allowed Frequently): coconut, flax; AVOID: borage seed, canola, cod liver.

Nuts and Seeds

Nuts and seeds are a secondary source of protein for Blood Type O. Walnuts are highly recommended, as they are known to be helpful in regulating insulin. Overall, however, your intake of vegetable proteins such as nuts, seeds, and beans should be limited to the portions and frequencies recommended, because they do not build active tissue mass or burn calories as efficiently as lean meats, fowl, and fish.

BLOOD TYPE O: NUTS AND SEEDS			
Portion: Whole (handful); Nut Butters (2 tblsp)			
	African	Caucasian	Asian
Secretor	2–5	2–5	2–4
Non-Secretor	5–7	5–7	5–7
			Times per week

SUPER BENEFICIAL	BENEFICIAL	NEUTRAL: Allowed Frequently	NEUTRAL: Allowed Infrequently	AVOID
Filbert (hazelnut)	Pumpkin seed	Almond	Sesame butter (tahini)	Beechnut
Flax (linseed)		Almond butter	Sesame seed	Brazil nut
Walnut		Almond cheese	Safflower seed	Cashew
		Almond milk		Chestnut
		Butternut		Litchi
		Hickory		Peanut
		Macadamia		Peanut butter
		Pecan		Pistachio
		Pignolia (pine nut)		Poppy seed
				Sunflower butter
				Sunflower seed

Special Variants: *Non-Secretor* NEUTRAL (Allowed Frequently): flax (linseed); AVOID: almond cheese, almond milk, safflower seed.

Beans and Legumes

Essentially a carnivore when it comes to protein requirements, Blood Type O can benefit from proteins found in some beans and legumes, although several of them contain problematic lectins. Given the choice, get your protein from animal foods.

BLOOD TYPE O: BEANS AND LEGUMES			
Portion: 1 cup (cooked)			
	African	Caucasian	Asian
Secretor	1–3	1–3	2–4
Non-Secretor	0–2	0–3	2–4
		Times per week	

SUPER BENEFICIAL	BENEFICIAL	NEUTRAL: Allowed Frequently	NEUTRAL: Allowed Infrequently	AVOID
Bean (green/ snap/ string)	Adzuki bean	Black bean	Soy milk	Copper bean
Fava (broad) bean	Black-eyed pea	Cannellini bean		Kidney bean
Northern bean		Garbanzo (chickpea)		Lentil (all)
		Jicama bean		Navy bean
		Lima bean		Pinto bean
		Miso		Tamarind bean
		Mung bean/ sprout		
		Pea (green/ pod/snow)		
		Tempeh		
		Soy bean		
		Soy cheese		
		Tofu		
		White bean		

Special Variants: *Non-Secretor* NEUTRAL (Allowed Frequently): adzuki bean, black-eyed pea, lentil (all), pinto bean; AVOID: fava (broad) bean, garbanzo, soy (all).

Grains and Starches

Grains and starches are the Achilles' heel of Blood Type O. You tend to do poorly on corn, wheat, sorghum, barley, and many of their by-products (sweeteners, etc.). These common grains have a very pronounced effect on increasing body fat and promoting insulin resistance in Blood Type O, and other grains are by no means necessary in your diet.

BLOOD TYPE O: GRAINS AND STARCHES			
Portion: ½ cup dry (grains or pastas); 1 muffin; 2 slices of bread			
	African	**Caucasian**	**Asian**
Secretor	1–6	1–6	1–6
Non-Secretor	0–3	0–3	0–3
		Times per week	

SUPER BENEFICIAL	BENEFICIAL	NEUTRAL: Allowed Frequently	NEUTRAL: Allowed Infrequently	AVOID
	Essene bread (Manna)	Amaranth Ezekiel 4:9 bread Kamut Quinoa Spelt (flour/ products) Spelt (whole) Tapioca Teff	Buck-wheat Millet Oat bran Oat flour Oatmeal Rice (whole) Rice (wild) Rice cake Rice flour Rice milk Rye (whole) Rye (flour/ products)	Barley Cornmeal Couscous Grits Popcorn Sorghum Wheat (re-fined/un-bleached) Wheat (semolina) Wheat (white flour) Wheat (whole) Wheat bran Wheat germ

SUPER BENEFICIAL	BENEFICIAL	NEUTRAL: Allowed Frequently	NEUTRAL: Allowed Infrequently	AVOID
	100% sprouted grain products (except Essene)		Soba noodles (100% buck-wheat) Soy flour/ products	

Special Variants: *Non-Secretor* AVOID: buckwheat, oat (all), soba noodles (100% buckwheat), soy flour/products, spelt (whole), spelt (flour/products), tapioca.

Vegetables

Vegetables provide a rich source of antioxidants and fiber, and several—especially mushrooms, broccoli, and greens—support insulin regulation. Many vegetables recommended for Blood Type O are also rich in potassium, which helps lower extracellular water in the body (edema), while raising intracellular water. Mushrooms are extremely beneficial for Blood Type O diabetics. Research shows that the mushroom lectin (*Agaricus bisporus*) stimulates insulin release from the pancreas, and aids proper insulin utilization. For Blood Type O, this is especially true of abalone, enoki, maitake, oyster, portobello, and straw varieties.

The common domestic white mushroom is referred to as "silver dollar." An item's value also applies to its juice, unless otherwise noted.

BLOOD TYPE O: VEGETABLES			
Portion: 1 cup, prepared (cooked or raw)			
	African	Caucasian	Asian
Secretor Beneficials	Unlimited	Unlimited	Unlimited
Secretor Neutrals	2–5	2–5	2–5
Non-Secretor Beneficials	Unlimited	Unlimited	Unlimited
Non-Secretor Neutrals	2–3	2–3	2–3
	Times per day		

SUPER BENEFICIAL	BENEFICIAL	NEUTRAL: Allowed Frequently	NEUTRAL: Allowed Infrequently	AVOID
Beet greens	Artichoke	Arugula	Brussels sprout	Alfalfa sprouts
Broccoli	Dandelion	Asparagus	Cabbage	Aloe
Chicory	Horse-radish	Asparagus pea	Olive (Greek/ green/ Spanish)	Cauliflower
Collard	Kohlrabi	Bamboo shoot		Corn
Escarole	Lettuce (romaine)	Bean (green/ snap/ string)	Yam	Cucumber
Kale				Leek
Mushroom (maitake)	Mushroom (abalone/ enoki/ oyster/ porto-bello/ straw/ tree ear)	Beet		Mushroom (shiitake/ silver-dollar)
Seaweed		Bok choy		Mustard greens
Spinach		Carrot		Olive (black)
Swiss chard	Okra	Celeriac		Potato
	Onion (all)	Celery		
	Parsnip	Chili pepper		
	Potato (sweet)	Daikon radish		
	Pumpkin	Eggplant		
	Turnip	Endive		
		Fennel		
		Fiddlehead fern		
		Garlic		
		Lettuce (except romaine)		
		Pea (green/ pod/ snow)		
		Peppers (all)		
		Poi		

SUPER BENEFICIAL	BENEFICIAL	NEUTRAL: Allowed Frequently	NEUTRAL: Allowed Infrequently	AVOID
		Radicchio		
		Radish/ sprouts		
		Rappini (broccoli rabe)		
		Rutabaga		
		Scallion		
		Shallot		
		Squash		
		Tomato		
		Water chestnut		
		Watercress		
		Zucchini		

Special Variants: *Non-Secretor* BENEFICIAL: carrot, fiddlehead fern, garlic; NEUTRAL (Allowed Frequently): lettuce (romaine), mushroom (except shiitake), mustard greens, parsnip, potato (sweet), turnip; AVOID: Brussels sprout, cabbage, eggplant, olive (all), poi.

Fruits and Fruit Juices

Eating plenty of fruit favorable to Blood Type O can encourage weight loss by tempering the effects of insulin. Also, fruits can help shift the balance of water in the body from high extracellular concentrations (edema) to high intracellular concentrations. Many fruits, such as pineapple, are rich in enzymes that can help reduce inflammation and encourage proper water balance. An item's value also applies to its juice, unless otherwise noted.

BLOOD TYPE O: FRUITS			
Portion: 1 cup			
	African	Caucasian	Asian
Secretor	2–4	3–5	3–5
Non-Secretor	1–3	1–3	1–3
		Times per day	

SUPER BENEFICIAL	BENEFICIAL	NEUTRAL: Allowed Frequently	NEUTRAL: Allowed Infrequently	AVOID
Blueberry	Banana	Boysen-berry	Apple	Asian pear
Pineapple	Cherry	Breadfruit	Apricot	Avocado
Plum	Elderberry	Canang melon	Currant	Bitter melon
Prune	(dark blue/ purple)	Casaba melon	Date	Blackberry
	Fig (fresh/ dried)	Christmas melon	Grapes (all)	Cantaloupe
	Guava	Cranberry	Quince	Coconut
	Mango	Crenshaw melon	Raisin	Honeydew
		Dewberry	Star fruit (caram-bola)	Kiwi
		Goose-berry	Strawberry	Orange
		Grapefruit		Plantain
		Kumquat		Tangerine
		Lemon		
		Lime		
		Logan-berry		
		Mulberry		
		Musk-melon		
		Nectarine		
		Papaya		

SUPER BENEFICIAL	BENEFICIAL	NEUTRAL: Allowed Frequently	NEUTRAL: Allowed Infrequently	AVOID
		Peach		
		Pear		
		Persian melon		
		Persimmon		
		Pomegranate		
		Prickly pear		
		Raspberry		
		Sago palm		
		Spanish melon		
		Watermelon		
		Youngberry		

Special Variants: *Non-Secretor* BENEFICIAL: avocado, pomegranate, prickly pear; NEUTRAL (Allowed Frequently): elderberry (dark blue/purple); AVOID: apple, apricot, date, strawberry.

Spices/Condiments/Sweeteners

Many spices have mild to moderate medicinal properties, often through their influence on the balance of bacteria in the lower intestine, enabling the proper digestion and metabolism of foods. Many common food adddadditives, such as guar gum and carrageenan, should be avoided, as they can enhance the effects of lectins found in other foods.

SUPER BENEFICIAL	BENEFICIAL	NEUTRAL: Allowed Frequently	NEUTRAL: Allowed Infrequently	AVOID
Fenugreek Turmeric	Carob Ginger Horse- radish Parsley Pepper (cayenne) Seaweed	Agar Allspice Almond extract Anise Basil Bay leaf Bergamot Caraway Cardamom Chervil Chili powder Chive Cilantro (coriander leaf) Cinnamon Clove Coriander Cream of tartar Cumin Dill Garlic Gelatin, plain Lecithin Licorice root Marjoram Mayon- naise	Apple pectin Arrowroot Barley malt Chocolate Honey Ketchup Maple syrup Molasses Molasses (black- strap) Rice syrup Senna Soy sauce Sucanat Sugar (brown/ white)	Aspartame Caper Carrageenan Cornstarch Corn syrup Dextrose Fructose Guarana Gums (acacia/ Arabic/ guar) Juniper Mace Malto- dextrin MSG Nutmeg Pepper (black/ white) Vinegar (except apple cider) Worcester- shire sauce

SUPER BENEFICIAL	BENEFICIAL	NEUTRAL: Allowed Frequently	NEUTRAL: Allowed Infrequently	AVOID
		Mint (all)		
		Miso		
		Mustard (dry)		
		Oregano		
		Paprika		
		Pepper (peppercorn/ red flakes)		
		Rosemary		
		Saffron		
		Sage		
		Savory		
		Sea salt		
		Stevia		
		Tamari (wheat-free)		
		Tamarind		
		Tarragon		
		Thyme		
		Vanilla		
		Vegetable glycerine		
		Vinegar (apple cider)		
		Wintergreen		

SUPER BENEFICIAL	BENEFICIAL	NEUTRAL: Allowed Frequently	NEUTRAL: Allowed Infrequently	AVOID
		Yeast (baker's/ brewer's)		

Special Variants: *Non-Secretor* BENEFICIAL: basil, bay leaf, licorice root,* oregano, saffron, tarragon, yeast (brewer's); NEUTRAL (Allowed Frequently): carob, MSG, nutmeg, turmeric; AVOID: agar, barley malt, cinnamon, honey, maple syrup, mayonnaise, miso, rice syrup, sage, soy sauce, stevia, sucanat, sugar (brown/white), tamari (wheatfree), vanilla, vinegar (apple cider).

*Do not use if you have high blood pressure.

Herbal Teas

Herbal teas can provide medicinal benefits and are excellent replacements for caffeinated drinks such as coffee, cola, and black tea.

SUPER BENEFICIAL	BENEFICIAL	NEUTRAL: Allowed Frequently	NEUTRAL: Allowed Infrequently	AVOID
Dandelion	Chickweed	Catnip		Alfalfa
Fenugreek	Hops	Chamomile		Aloe
Ginger	Linden	Dong Quai		Burdock
	Mulberry	Elder		Coltsfoot
	Peppermint	Ginseng		Corn silk
	Rosehip	Hawthorn		Echinacea
	Sarsaparilla	Horehound		Gentian
	Slippery elm	Licorice		Goldenseal
		Mullein		Red clover
		Raspberry leaf		Rhubarb
		Senna		Shepherd's purse
		Skullcap		St. John's wort

SUPER BENEFICIAL	BENEFICIAL	NEUTRAL: Allowed Frequently	NEUTRAL: Allowed Infrequently	AVOID
		Spearmint Valerian Vervain White birch White oak bark Yarrow		Strawberry leaf Yellow dock

Miscellaneous Beverages

Avoid or limit alcohol (except red wine), which can promote insulin resistance. Coffee can trigger a hypoglycemic reaction.

SUPER BENEFICIAL	BENEFICIAL	NEUTRAL: Allowed Frequently	NEUTRAL: Allowed Infrequently	AVOID
Tea (green)	Seltzer Soda (club)	Wine (red)		Beer Coffee (reg/decaf) Liquor Soda, (cola/diet/misc.) Tea, black (reg/decaf) Wine (white)

Supplement Protocols

THE DIET FOR BLOOD TYPE O offers abundant quantities of important nutrients. It's vital to get as many nutrients as possible from fresh foods, and to use supplements only to fill in the minor blanks in your diet. The following Supplement Protocols are designed for pre-diabetic metabolic enhancement, diabetes management, and support for treatment of diabetic complications. For information about specially formulated, blood type–specific supplements, visit our Web site, www.dadamo.com.

Note: If you are taking insulin or diabetes medications, or are being treated for a related condition, consult your doctor before taking any supplements.

Blood Type O: Pre-Diabetes/ Metabolic Enhancement Protocol

For support of overall metabolic health and blood sugar regulation		
SUPPLEMENT	**ACTION**	**DOSAGE**
High-potency multi-vitamin, preferably blood type–specific	Nutritional support	As directed
High-potency mineral complex, preferably blood type–specific	Nutritional support	As directed
Larch arabinogalactan	Promotes intestinal health; excellent fiber source	1 tablespoon, twice daily, in juice or water
Probiotic	Promotes intestinal health	1–2 capsules, twice daily
Bladderwrack	Improves metabolic health, regulates thyroid activity, and promotes weight loss	1–2 capsules daily, away from meals
Chromium	Helps metabolize carbohydrates	50 mcg, once daily, or 1 teaspoon chromium-containing brewer's yeast

Blood Type O: Type 1 Diabetes Adjunct

SUPPLEMENT	ACTION	DOSAGE
Quercetin	Prevents diabetic complications	300–600 mg, twice daily
Zinc	Prevents deficiency common to type 1 diabetics	25 mg daily

Blood Type O: Type 2 Diabetes Adjunct

SUPPLEMENT	ACTION	DOSAGE
Quercetin	Prevents diabetic complications, aids blood sugar regulation	300–600 mg, twice daily
Fenugreek	Lowers blood sugar, improves glucose tolerance	300–600 mg, twice daily
Asian ginseng	Stabilizes blood sugar and prevents post-meal hyperglycemia	100–300 mg, 40 minutes before eating (avoid if you have high blood pressure)

Blood Type O: Diabetic Complications Adjunct

SUPPLEMENT	ACTION	DOSAGE
Alpha-lipoic acid	Improves diabetic neuropathy and reduces pain	100–300 mg, twice daily
Dandelion (*Taraxacum officinale*)	Reduces edema	250 mg capsule daily, or fresh in salad or tea
Stinging nettle root (*Urtica dioica*)	Reduces edema	500 mg, 1–2 times daily, away from meals

SUPPLEMENT	ACTION	DOSAGE
Cayenne (*Capsicum frutescens*)	Relieves numbness and pain in the extremities associated with diabetic neuropathy	In a topical cream, 3–4 times daily

The Exercise Component

BLOOD TYPE O benefits tremendously from brisk regular exercise that taxes the cardiovascular and musculoskeletal systems. Your goal should be to develop as much active tissue mass as possible; this is the key to your metabolic fitness.

Exercise is also crucial to a well-regulated chemical-release system. The act of physical exercise releases a swarm of neurotransmitter activity that acts as a tonic for the entire system. More than any other blood type, Blood Type Os require regular, high-intensity physical exercise to maintain health and emotional balance. Below is a list of exercises that are recommended for Blood Type O, along with some general tips for making the most of your exercise program.

Build a balanced routine of both aerobic and strength-training activities from the following options:

EXERCISE	DURATION	FREQUENCY
Aerobics	40–60 minutes	3–4 x week
Weight training	30–45 minutes	3–4 x week
Running	40–45 minutes	3–4 x week
Calisthenics	30–45 minutes	3 x week
Treadmill	30 minutes	3 x week
Kickboxing	30–45 minutes	3 x week
Cycling	30 minutes	3 x week
Contact sports	60 minutes	2–3 x week
In-line/roller-skating	30 minutes	2–3 x week

Three Steps to Effective Exercise

1. Before you begin your aerobic exercise, warm up with a walk. Then perform some careful stretching movements to increase flexibility.
2. To achieve maximum cardiovascular benefits, work toward an elevated heart rate that is about 70 percent of your capacity. Once you reach the elevated rate, continue exercising to maintain that rate for twenty to thirty minutes. To calculate your maximum heart rate and performance level:
   - Subtract your age from 220.
   - Multiply the difference by .70 (or .60 if you are over sixty). This is the high end of your performance.
   - Multiply the remainder by .50. This is the low end of your performance.
3. Finish each aerobic session with a cool-down of at least five minutes, combining some careful stretching and flexibility movements with a relaxing walk.

Blood Type O Diabetes Diet Checklist

Eat small to moderate portions of high-quality, lean, organic ☐ meat several times a week for strength, energy, and efficient metabolism. Meat should be prepared medium to rare for the best health effects. If you charbroil, or cook meat well-done, use a marinade composed of healthy ingredients such as cherry juice, lemon juice, spices, and herbs.

Include regular portions of richly oiled cold-water fish. Fish ☐ oil helps counter inflammatory conditions, improves thyroid function, and boosts your metabolism.

Consume little or no dairy foods. They are difficult for you to ☐ digest.

Eliminate wheat and wheat-based products from your diet. ☐
They usually cause more problems than any other food for
Type Os. If you have digestive or weight problems, also elim-
inate oats.

Limit your intake of beans, as they are not a particularly good ☐
protein source for Type Os.

Eat lots of BENEFICIAL fruits and vegetables. ☐

Use BENEFICIAL and NEUTRAL nuts and dried fruits for snacks. ☐

If you need a daily dose of caffeine, replace coffee with green ☐
tea. It isn't acidic and has substantially less caffeine than coffee.

Avoid foods that are Type O red flags, especially wheat, corn, ☐
kidney beans, navy beans, lentils, peanuts, potatoes, and cau-
liflower.

Getting Started: The First Month

IF YOU ARE NEW to the Blood Type Diet and exercise plan, the following guidelines will introduce you to the Blood Type O regimen over
a period of one month. Follow these recommendations as closely as
possible, using a journal to record your progress and to write down your
personal experience with the diet. In addition to measurable factors—
such as weight loss, blood sugar regulation, and blood pressure—take
the time to note changes in energy levels, sleep patterns, mood, and
overall well-being. Over time you'll learn to manage your diet and exercise patterns to achieve the maximum results.

Week 1

Blood Type Diet and Supplements

- Cut back or eliminate your most harmful AVOID foods—wheat and dairy.
  These foods seriously interfere with proper metabolism.
- Include your most important BENEFICIAL foods at least five times this week.
  These include lean organic meat, seafood, and vegetables.

- Incorporate at least one SUPER BENEFICIAL food into your daily diet. For example, have a handful of walnuts as a snack, or throw some fresh blueberries into your morning cereal.

- If you're a coffee drinker, begin to wean yourself by cutting your daily consumption in half. Substitute a high-quality green tea, such as Itaru's Premium Green Tea, which is available from our Web site (see Appendix B).

- To improve blood sugar regulation, eat 5 to 6 small meals throughout the day, rather than 3 large meals. Never skip meals.

- Drink a cup of dandelion or fenugreek tea every evening.

- If you are taking insulin or diabetes medications, speak with your doctor before taking supplements; your dosages may need to be changed.

Exercise Regimen

- Plan to exercise at least 4 days this week, for 45 minutes each day.

  2 days: aerobic activity

  2 days: weights

- Use your journal to detail the time, activity, distance, rate, and amount of weight used. Note the repetitions used for each exercise.

▪ WEEK 1 SUCCESS STRATEGY ▪

Start slowly, giving yourself a chance to get used to the Blood Type O Diet. You'll have a much better chance of long-term success if you take some time to incorporate the Blood Type Diet recommendations into your daily life. I've found that the biggest indicator of failure is a rigid adherence to the plan from the first day on. I know you want to get moving and start seeing results. That's a positive goal. But patience is your friend if you want to make a permanent change in your diet and lifestyle.

Week 2

Blood Type Diet and Supplements

- Begin to eliminate the next level of AVOID foods—corn, potatoes, beans, and legumes.

- Eat at least one BENEFICIAL animal protein every day.

- Initially, it is best to avoid foods on the NEUTRAL: Allowed Infrequently list. After you have been on the diet for four weeks, you may begin to incorporate them 1–2 times a month.

- Continue to incorporate SUPER BENEFICIAL foods into your diet, at least twice a day.
- If you're a coffee drinker, continue to cut your coffee intake, replacing it with BENEFICIAL herbal teas or high-quality green tea, such as Itaru's Premium Green Tea.
- Continue to eat 5 to 6 small meals throughout the day, rather than 3 large meals.

Exercise Regimen

- Continue to exercise at least 4 days this week, for 45 minutes each day.

  2 days: aerobic activity

  2 days: weights
- If your work is sedentary, get in the habit of taking a couple of "movement" breaks during the day. Walk around the block or up and down stairs.

▪ WEEK 2 SUCCESS STRATEGY▪

Don't leave home without a quick snack tucked into your purse or briefcase to offset low blood sugar.

Suggestions:

- Super Smoothie in a Thermos, made with albumin-based protein powder (or whole boiled egg), 1 cup blueberries, 1 banana, and ½ cup pineapple juice
- Trail mix: walnuts, raisins, dried blueberries, dried cherries, dried pineapple

---

Week 3

Blood Type Diet and Supplements

- When you plan your meals for week 3, choose BENEFICIAL foods to replace NEUTRAL foods whenever possible. For example, choose lamb over chicken, or a plum instead of an apple.
- Eliminate all remaining AVOID foods.
- Liberally incorporate SUPER BENEFICIAL foods into your daily diet. For instance, slice mushrooms into salads or snack on walnuts.
- Completely wean yourself from coffee, substituting Itaru's Premium Green Tea.
- Continue to eat 5 to 6 small meals throughout the day, rather than 3 large meals.

- Drink a cup of licorice tea after meals to balance blood sugar. (Not for Type Os with high blood pressure.)

Exercise Regimen

- Continue to exercise at least 4 days this week, for 45 minutes each day.

  2 days: aerobic activity

  2 days: weights

- Add one day of unstructured exercise—walking, biking, swimming.

▪ WEEK 3 SUCCESS STRATEGY ▪

Fight carbohydrate cravings. If you crave any form of stimulants or carbohydrates, your serotonin levels are low, and your brain is demanding stimulants to raise your serotonin levels.

- Try a sip of vegetable glycerine between meals to cut down on your cravings. For women, low estrogen levels can produce carbohydrate craving. One or two capsules of the herb maca can help normalize your estrogen levels.

Week 4

Blood Type Diet and Supplements

- Continue at the week 3 level, focusing on SUPER BENEFICIAL and BENEFICIAL foods.

- Continue to eat 5 to 6 small meals throughout the day, rather than 3 large meals.

- Evaluate the first three weeks and make adjustments. If you have kept a detailed journal, you should have a clear idea wich eating patterns and foods have made the most profound difference—both positively and negatively.

Exercise Regimen

- Continue at the week 3 level.

- Evaluate your progress, referring to your journal. Determine which exercise regimen has worked for you, including time of day, setting, and activity level. Look for ways to improve your performance and endurance.

■ **WEEK 4 SUCCESS STRATEGY** ■

Combat exercise boredom:

- Find an exercise buddy. A brisk morning walk with a friend can reinvigorate your daily effort.
- Cross-train. Choose a different aerobic activity every third day.
- Challenge yourself with specific goals: time, endurance, or pace. Reward yourself when you reach your goals.
- Don't overtrain. It can lead to injuries and have a negative effect on blood sugar levels. The key is consistency.

FAQs: Blood Type O and Diabetes

Is it okay to drink a glass of wine with dinner?

Alcohol can lower blood glucose for eight to twelve hours after your last drink. Usually, if your blood glucose drops too low, the liver puts more glucose into the blood. (The liver has its own supply of glucose, called glycogen.) But when alcohol, a toxin, is in the body, the liver wants to get rid of it first. While the liver is taking care of the alcohol it may let blood glucose drop to dangerously low levels.

Alcohol can also elevate blood pressure and increase triglycerides. If you have diabetes-associated nerve damage or eye diseases, avoid all alcohol. Red wine should be preferred over white; it has less sugar, and the red pigments can help protect nerve and eye tissue from the effects of the diabetic process.

Why must coffee be avoided by Blood Type O diabetics?

There is strong evidence that even moderate amounts of caffeine can activate Blood Type O's sympathetic nervous system, resulting in a higher adrenaline release. Studies show that Type O individuals also take longer to clear adrenaline out of their systems. This adrenaline release mimics a condition of hypoglycemia, even when your blood sugar levels are not actually low. The primary symptoms include sweating, tremor, palpitations, sensation of hunger, restlessness, and anxiety. Other symptoms you might experience are caused by an insufficient supply of glucose to the brain, resulting in blurred vision, weakness, slurred speech, vertigo, and difficulties in concentration.

Shouldn't blood glucose levels go down after exercising? My glucose levels go up. What could be causing this?

Blood glucose levels usually do go down after exercise, providing that the body has adequate insulin on board for glucose utilization. If your blood glucose level is greater than 240 to 250 mg/dL before exercising, the exercise will make your blood glucose go higher. Exercise can affect your blood glucose for up to forty-eight hours afterward. During exercise, if glucose levels are lower before exertion, the body will pull from stored glycogen in the liver and muscles that is released to provide energy. Usually after twenty to thirty minutes of exercise these glucose reserves are depleted, and if you overexercise, you may see a slight rise in levels. After a sustained period of exercise, at appropriate levels, your blood sugar should drop.

Can I use the glycemic index on the Blood Type Diet?

The glycemic index measures the amount of carbohydrates in foods. However, it is not *how much* carbohydrate, but *what kind* of carbohydrate, that makes the difference. The glycemic index is only one aspect of food analysis. The Blood Type Diet goes beyond the general observation of a food's effect on blood sugar levels, evaluating the kinds of sugars present, any lectin activity, the relative amount of beneficial substances, and other blood type–mediated issues. For instance, pineapple juice contains anti-inflammatory and protein-digestive enzymes. Black cherries are high in antioxidant compounds. In contrast, apples and oranges have much lower glycemic index ratings than pineapple, but apples contain a lectin affecting Type O non-secretors and have little to offer aside from fruit pectin, while oranges promote harmful polyamine production. Many foods containing Blood Type O reactive lectins that can interfere with proper insulin function are themselves rather low on the glycemic index. The key is to evaluate the effects of the whole food on the entire body of each individual. In sum, go with your food list.

Are there any safe sugar substitutes for Blood Type O?

Vegetable glycerine, widely available in health-food stores, has beneficial effects on your body's ability to release energy from the food you eat and can be used in place of any sweetener you now employ.

Why is soda water or seltzer beneficial for Type O?

Room temperature seltzer helps to regulate the hormone gastrin, which acts on the appetite center. A glass of room-temperature seltzer water about twenty minutes before a meal not only aids digestion but helps curb your appetite as well.

I am a Type O with Hashimoto's thyroiditis. Will this make me more liable to get diabetes?

Blood Type O individuals have a special susceptibility to thyroid problems, caused by either an overproduction (hyperthyroidism) or underproduction (hypothyroidism) of the thyroid hormone thyroxine. Hashimoto's thyroiditis is a condition caused by an underproduction of thyroxine. It can produce weight gain, fluid retention, and fatigue, which are all triggers in the development of diabetes. Your best course of action is to follow the diet and exercise guidelines for Blood Type O. Many Type Os have successfully dealt with their Hashimoto's thyroiditis simply by following the low-grain Type O Diet.

I have been diagnosed with type 2 diabetes. Since I began taking medication to control it, I have been gaining weight, and my stomach feels bloated and distended. This doesn't seem to be an improvement. Is there any way I can avoid these results?

When you begin improving your blood sugar control, it's not unusual to experience weight gain. That's because the glucose is being assimilated rather than spilling out through your urine. If you are following the diet for Blood Type O and exercising vigorously, the weight gain and water retention will be temporary. It is especially important not to skip meals or severely cut calories. These strategies will only encourage more weight gain.

My Blood Type O son has been diagnosed with type 1 diabetes. Is it safe for him to exercise the way he did before? He has always been very active in sports.

Encourage your son to continue his activities. Physical exercise will improve his condition and his general feeling of well-being by regulating his blood sugar. Team sports are excellent for Blood Type O children, who tend to be extroverted. Continuing team activities that he enjoyed before his diagnosis will support his sense that he fits in, instead of allowing his disease to dominate and isolate him. Like so many other aspects of diabetes management, the key is planning ahead. Since vigorous exercise can drive blood sugar levels down, make sure your son always has a quick snack ready. Pack some trail mix, a piece of fruit, or a small carton of beneficial juice in his knapsack.

A Final Word

IN SUMMARY, the secret to fighting diabetes with the Blood Type O Diet involves:

1. Increasing active tissue mass (calorie-burning tissue) by adhering to a diet that is animal protein–based.
2. Minimizing consumption of the insulin-mimicking lectins, most abundant in grains, such as wheat and corn.
3. Increasing circulatory efficiency, lowering adrenaline, and minimizing arterial damage by adopting a vigorous exercise program.
4. Using supplements intelligently to block the effect of insulin-mimicking lectins, providing antioxidant support, and protect delicate nerve tissue from destruction.

Blood Type

A

ROM A PURELY STATISTICAL STANDPOINT, BLOOD TYPE A has a higher risk than the other blood types of both type 1 and type 2 diabetes. This association has been confirmed in several large independent studies examining and tracking literally thousands of people.

Blood Type A individuals are also more likely to have cardiovascular complications due to diabetes, as well as complications related to blood clotting. In many ways, Blood Type A is the exact opposite of Blood Type O when it comes to metabolism. While animal protein speeds up the Blood Type O metabolic rate and makes it more efficient, it has a very different effect on Blood Type A. Many meat-eating Blood Type As report feeling fatigued and lacking energy, especially when they engage in aerobic exercise and restrict complex carbohydrates. They also complain of fluid retention, because they are unable to properly digest high-protein foods. While Blood Type O burns meat as fuel, Blood Type A tends to store meat as fat.

Blood Type A Weight Profile

Weight Gain		Weight Loss	
FOOD	**MECHANISM**	**FOOD**	**MECHANISM**
Red meat	Poorly digested and stored as fat	Soy	Improves insulin metabolism
Kidney, lima beans	Promote insulin resistance and block digestive enzymes	Seafood, fish oils	Improve insulin metabolism and prevent fluid retention
Dairy	Creates insulin resistance	Broccoli, spinach	Aid efficient metabolism
Wheat	Creates insulin resistance and impairs calorie utilization	Mushrooms	Improve insulin metabolism
Corn, potatoes	Create insulin resistance	Pineapple	Improves insulin metabolism and aids digestion

The currently popular high-protein diets can be folly for Blood Type A. These diets are based on the premise that carbohydrates in the diet elevate insulin levels and cause weight gain. Some use the glycemic index, said to be the rate at which certain foods spike insulin production. I've always suspected that these diets have achieved their following because of Blood Type Os, for whom high-protein diets are beneficial. Anecdotally, I've found this to be true among my patients and those who have reported their experiences on my Web site. However, Blood Type A individuals usually do very poorly on high-protein diets. Like most reductionistic approaches, the glycemic index doesn't take into account additional factors, which may influence some people's ability to metabolize certain foods. Many foods with high glycemic ratings also happen to be rich sources of insulin-mimicking lectins. Here we're evaluating individual foods, not entire categories of foods. With discriminating tools, such as blood types, we now know why a food may enhance insulin in one person, yet inhibit it in the next.

When Blood Type A diabetics overconsume meat, it increases their overall cholesterol as well as their LDL cholesterol. In combination with their general tendency to have blood that clots more easily, these factors can cause Blood Type A diabetics to have a greater risk of developing cardiovascular and arterial complications from diabetes.

The Diabetes-Stress Factor

BLOOD TYPE AS who struggle with low metabolism and weight gain have another challenge—the effects of high levels of the stress hormone cortisol. As we described earlier, cortisol promotes insulin resistance and hormonal imbalance.

With Blood Type A's added difficulties due to the stress-cortisol connection, you may need to work a bit harder to stay energized. Try to establish a regular sleep schedule and adhere to it as closely as possible. When you have a normal sleep-wake rhythm, cortisol levels normalize as well. During the day, schedule at least two breaks of twenty minutes each for complete relaxation. Combat sleep disturbances with regular exercise and a relaxing pre-bedtime routine. A light snack before bedtime will help raise your blood sugar levels and improve sleep. Most important, be attentive to the factors in your daily life that elevate your stress levels. When you take steps to eliminate stressors, you are doing more than simply improving your mood. You're protecting your health.

Special Risks for Non-Secretors

BLOOD TYPE A non-secretors are at greater risk of developing diabetes and of developing complications from diabetes.

From a statistical standpoint alone, non-secretors are three times more likely than secretors to become diabetic. Overall, Blood Type A non-secretors have a higher risk of all conditions associated with Metabolic Syndrome, including high cholesterol, hypertension, and insulin resistance.

Research shows that several of the Blood Type A risk factors become magnified when you are a non-secretor. The activity of intestinal alkaline phosphatase, which is involved in the breakdown of protein and fat, is already low in Blood Type A, and is even lower in Blood Type A non-secretors. If you are a Type A non-secretor, your alkaline phosphatase activity is only about 20 percent of that of secretors. Being a non-secretor also has an impact on blood-clotting ability. Blood Type A tends to have elevated levels of certain clotting factors, contributing to your risk for heart disease and thrombosis. If you are also a non-secretor, your clotting factors are raised even higher.

Taken together, these factors can make a big difference for a Blood Type A individual, so it's important that you find out your secretor status. (See Appendix B for information about ordering a saliva test.)

Blood Type A: The Foods

THE BLOOD TYPE A Diabetes Diet is specifically adapted for the prevention and management of diabetes. The new category, **Super Beneficial**, highlights powerful diabetes-fighting foods for Blood Type A. The **Neutral** category has also been adjusted to de-emphasize foods that can cause problems for diabetics. Foods designated **Neutral: Allowed Infrequently** should be minimized or avoided, depending on your condition. Eat these foods no more than once or twice a month.

Your secretor status can influence your ability to fully digest and metabolize certain foods, so some adjustments in the values are included for non-secretors. If you do not know your secretor type, the odds are that you can safely use the "secretor" values, since the majority of the population (80 percent) are secretors. However, I urge you to get tested, since the variations are important for non-secretors who want to maximize the effectiveness of the Blood Type Diet.

The food charts are divided into three sections. The top of the chart suggests the average portion size and quantity per week or day, according to secretor status. These recommendations do *not* apply to the category **Neutral: Allowed Infrequently;** those foods should be consumed sparingly (0–2 times a month). For some foods the charts

Food Values

SUPER BENEFICIAL	Foods that are known to have specific disease-fighting qualities for your blood type.
BENEFICIAL	Foods with components that enhance the metabolic, immune, or structural health of your blood type.
NEUTRAL: **Allowed Frequently**	Foods that normally have no direct blood type effect but supply a variety of nutrients necessary for a healthful diet.
NEUTRAL: **Allowed Infrequently**	Foods that normally have no blood type effect but may impede your progress when consumed regularly.
AVOID	Foods with components that are harmful to your blood type.

also indicate differences in frequency based on ethnic heritage. It has been my experience that this factor has an impact on the individual's ability to fully digest certain foods. For the purposes of blood type food choices, persons of Hispanic heritage should follow the recommendations for Caucasians, and North American Native peoples should follow the recommendations for Asians.

The middle section of the chart provides the food values. The bottom section lists variants based on secretor status.

For your convenience, we have included a number of product names, such as ketchup, Worcestershire sauce, and Ezekiel bread. However, bear in mind that commercial formulations vary among brands and regions. Even though a product may be listed as okay for you, always check its ingredients; do not use products that contain **Avoid** ingredients for your blood type. Of course, you may choose to make your own version of commercial products such as bread and mayonnaise, using ingredients that suit your blood type. There are hundreds of delicious recipes for every blood type available on our Web site (www.dadamo.com) and in the book *Cook Right 4 Your Type: The Practical Kitchen Companion to* Eat Right 4 Your Type.

Meat/Poultry

Blood Type A lacks some of the enzymes and stomach acids needed to effectively digest animal protein. For this reason you should derive most of your protein from nonmeat sources. Higher animal protein can aggravate the Type A tendency toward accelerated blood clotting, which can amplify the damage to arteries caused by the diabetic process. When you do eat meat or fowl, stick to small portions. Choose only the highest quality (preferably grass-fed) chemical-, antibiotic-, and pesticide-free, low-fat meats and poultry.

Non-secretors have a slight edge in digesting animal protein.

BLOOD TYPE A: MEAT/POULTRY			
Portion: 4–6 oz (men); 2–5 oz (women and children)			
	African	Caucasian	Asian
Secretor	0–2	0–3	0–3
Non-Secretor	2–5	2–4	2–3
		Times per week	

SUPER BENEFICIAL	BENEFICIAL	NEUTRAL: Allowed Frequently	NEUTRAL: Allowed Infrequently	AVOID
		Chicken		All commercially processed meat
		Cornish hen		Bacon/Ham/Pork
		Grouse		Beef
		Guinea hen		Buffalo
		Ostrich		Duck
		Squab		Goat
		Turkey		Goose
				Heart (beef)
				Horse

SUPER BENEFICIAL	BENEFICIAL	NEUTRAL: Allowed Frequently	NEUTRAL: Allowed Infrequently	AVOID
				Lamb
				Liver (calf)
				Mutton
				Partridge
				Pheasant
				Quail
				Rabbit
				Squirrel
				Sweetbreads
				Turtle
				Veal
				Venison

Special Variants: *Non-Secretor* BENEFICIAL: turkey; NEUTRAL (Allowed Frequently): duck, goat, goose, lamb, mutton, partridge, pheasant, quail, rabbit, turtle.

Fish/Seafood

Fish and seafood represent a nutrient-rich source of protein for Blood Type A. Because of this, fish is probably the best food for building active tissue mass. Many kinds of fish are rich in omega series fatty acids, which can help control blood sugar and lower the risk of cardiovascular disease.

BLOOD TYPE A: FISH/SEAFOOD			
Portion: 4–6 oz (men); 2–5 oz (women and children)			
	African	Caucasian	Asian
Secretor	1–3	1–3	1–3
Non-Secretor	2–5	2–5	2–4
		Times per week	

SUPER BENEFICIAL	BENEFICIAL	NEUTRAL: Allowed Frequently	NEUTRAL: Allowed Infrequently	AVOID
Cod	Carp	Abalone		Anchovy
Red snapper	Mackerel	Bass (sea)		Barracuda
Salmon	Monkfish	Bullhead		Bass (bluegill/ striped)
Sardine	Perch (silver/ yellow)	Butterfish		
Trout (rainbow)		Chub		Beluga
	Pickerel	Croaker		Bluefish
	Pollock	Cusk		Catfish
	Snail (*Helix pomatia*/ escargot)	Drum		Caviar (sturgeon)
		Halfmoon fish		Clam
	Trout (sea)	Mahi-mahi		Conch
	Whitefish	Mullet		Crab
	Whiting	Muskel- lunge		Crayfish
		Orange roughy		Eel
		Parrot fish		Flounder
		Perch (white)		Frog
		Pike		Gray sole
		Pompano		Grouper
		Porgy		Haddock
		Rosefish		Hake
		Sailfish		Halibut
		Salmon roe		Harvest fish
		Scrod		Herring (fresh/ pickled/ smoked)
		Shark		
		Smelt		Lobster
		Sturgeon		Mussels
		Sucker		Octopus
		Sunfish		Opaleye
				Oyster

SUPER BENEFICIAL	BENEFICIAL	NEUTRAL: Allowed Frequently	NEUTRAL: Allowed Infrequently	AVOID
		Swordfish		Salmon (smoked)
		Tilapia		Scallop
		Trout (brook)		Scup
		Tuna		Shad
		Weakfish		Shrimp
		Yellowtail		Sole
				Squid (calamari)
				Tilefish

Special Variants: *Non-Secretor* BENEFICIAL: chub, cusk, drum, halfmoon fish, harvest fish, mullet, muskellunge, perch (white), rosefish, sailfish, sucker, swordfish, trout (brook); NEUTRAL (Allowed Frequently): anchovy, bass (bluegill), beluga, bluefish, caviar (sturgeon), flounder, frog, gray sole, grouper, haddock, hake, halibut, herring (fresh), mussels, octopus, opaleye, scallops, scup, shad, tilefish.

Dairy/Eggs

Dairy products can be used in small quantities by Blood Type A. Be especially cautious if you suffer from recurrent sinus infections or colds, since dairy products can be mucus-forming for Blood Type A. In small quantities, eggs can serve as a complementary protein and are an excellent source of docosahexaenoic acid (DHA). Do your best to find eggs and dairy products that meet organic standards.

BLOOD TYPE A: EGGS			
Portion: 1 egg			
	African	Caucasian	Asian
Secretor	1–3	1–3	1–3
Non-Secretor	2–3	2–5	2–4
		Times per week	

BLOOD TYPE A: MILK AND YOGURT

Portion: 4–6 oz (men); 2–5 oz (women and children)

	African	Caucasian	Asian
Secretor	0–1	1–3	0–3
Non-Secretor	0–1	1–2	0–2
		Times per week	

BLOOD TYPE A: CHEESE

Portion: 3 oz (men); 2 oz (women and children)

	African	Caucasian	Asian
Secretor	0–2	1–3	0–2
Non-Secretor	0	0–1	0–1
		Times per week	

SUPER BENEFICIAL	BENEFICIAL	NEUTRAL: Allowed Frequently	NEUTRAL: Allowed Infrequently	AVOID
		Egg (chicken/ duck/ goose/ quail)	Feta	American cheese
		Farmer cheese	Goat cheese	Blue cheese
		Ghee (clarified butter)	Milk (goat)	Brie
		Kefir	Sour cream	Butter
		Mozzarella		Buttermilk
		Paneer		Camembert
		Ricotta		Casein
		Yogurt		Cheddar
				Colby
				Cottage cheese
				Cream cheese
				Edam
				Emmenthal

SUPER BENEFICIAL	BENEFICIAL	NEUTRAL: Allowed Frequently	NEUTRAL: Allowed Infrequently	AVOID
				Gouda
				Gruyère
				Half-and-half
				Ice cream
				Jarlsberg
				Milk (cow)
				Monterey Jack
				Muenster
				Neufchâtel
				Parmesan
				Provolone
				Sherbet
				Swiss cheese
				Whey

Special Variants: *Non-Secretor* NEUTRAL (Allowed Frequently): cottage cheese, whey; AVOID: milk (goat), sour cream.

Oils

In general, Blood Type A does best on monounsaturated oils (such as olive oil) and oils rich in omega series fatty acids (such as flax oil).

BLOOD TYPE A: OILS			
Portion: 1 tblsp			
	African	Caucasian	Asian
Secretor	5–8	5–8	5–8
Non-Secretor	3–7	3–7	3–6
	Times per week		

SUPER BENEFICIAL	BENEFICIAL	NEUTRAL: Allowed Frequently	NEUTRAL: Allowed Infrequently	AVOID
Flax (linseed)	Black currant seed Olive	Almond Borage seed	Canola	Castor Coconut Corn
	Walnut	Cod liver Evening primrose Safflower Sesame Soy Sunflower Wheat germ		Cottonseed Peanut

Special Variants: *Non-Secretor* BENEFICIAL: cod liver, sesame; NEUTRAL (Allowed Frequently): peanut; AVOID: safflower.

Nuts and Seeds

Nuts and seeds can serve as an important secondary source of protein for Blood Type A. Walnuts and peanuts can aid in blood sugar regulation. Flaxseeds are particularly rich in lignans, which can help lower intestinal toxicity.

BLOOD TYPE A: NUTS AND SEEDS			
Portion: Whole (handful); Nut Butters (2 tblsp)			
	African	Caucasian	Asian
Secretor	4–7	4–7	4–7
Non-Secretor	5–7	5–7	5–7
		Times per week	

SUPER BENEFICIAL	BENEFICIAL	NEUTRAL: Allowed Frequently	NEUTRAL: Allowed Infrequently	AVOID
Flax (linseed) Peanut Peanut butter Walnut (black/ English)	Pumpkin seed	Almond Almond butter Almond cheese Almond milk Beechnut Butternut Chestnut Filbert (hazel-nut) Hickory nut Litchi Macadamia nut Pecan Pignolia (pine nut) Poppy seed Sunflower butter Sunflower seed	Safflower seed Sesame butter (tahini) Sesame seed	Brazil nut Cashew Pistachio

Special Variants: *Non-Secretor* AVOID: safflower seed, sunflower seed.

Beans and Legumes

Blood Type A thrives on vegetable proteins found in many beans and legumes, although some beans contain problem lectins. In general, this category, along with appropriate choices of seafood, is more than sufficient to build active tissue mass for Blood Type A. The BENEFICIAL and SUPER BENEFICIAL beans are all excellent sources of essential amino acids, and are known to aid in blood sugar regulation.

BLOOD TYPE A: BEANS AND LEGUMES			
Portion: 1 cup (cooked)			
	African	Caucasian	Asian
Secretor	5–7	5–7	5–7
Non-Secretor	3–5	3–5	3–5
			Times per week

SUPER BENEFICIAL	BENEFICIAL	NEUTRAL: Allowed Frequently	NEUTRAL: Allowed Infrequently	AVOID
Bean (green/ snap/ string) Fava (broad) bean Miso Soy bean Soy cheese Soy milk Tempeh Tofu	Adzuki bean Black bean Black-eyed pea Lentil (all) Pinto bean	Cannellini bean Jicama bean Mung bean/ sprout Northern bean Pea (green/ pod/ snow White bean		Copper bean Garbanzo (chickpea) Kidney bean Lima bean Navy bean Tamarind bean

Special Variants: *Non-Secretor* NEUTRAL (Allowed Frequently): adzuki bean, black bean, black-eyed pea, copper bean, fava (broad) bean, kidney bean, navy bean, soy bean, soy cheese, soy milk, tempeh, tofu.

Grains and Starches

If you have a weight problem, are insulin-resistant, or have diabetes, limit your intake of wheat and corn; their lectins can exert an insulin-like effect, lowering active tissue mass and increasing total body fat.

The agglutinin in whole wheat can aggravate inflammatory conditions and lower active tissue mass. This lectin can often be milled out of the grain, or destroyed by sprouting.

BLOOD TYPE A: GRAINS AND STARCHES

Portion: ½ cup dry (grains or pastas); 1 muffin; 2 slices of bread

	African	Caucasian	Asian
Secretor	7–10	7–9	7–10
Non-Secretor	5–7	5–7	5–7
		Times per week	

SUPER BENEFICIAL	BENEFICIAL	NEUTRAL: Allowed Frequently	NEUTRAL: Allowed Infrequently	AVOID
	Amaranth	Barley	Cornmeal	Teff
	Buckwheat	Kamut	Couscous	Wheat bran
	Essene bread (Manna)	Quinoa	Grits	Wheat germ
	Ezekiel 4:9 bread	Rice (flour/ products)	Millet	
	Oat bran	Rice (wild)	Popcorn	
	Oat flour	Rice cake	Tapioca	
	Oatmeal	Rice milk	Wheat (whole)	
	Rice (whole)	Sorghum		
	Rice bran	Spelt (whole)		
	Rye (whole)	Spelt flour/ products		
	Soba noodles (100% buckwheat)	Wheat (re-fined/un-bleached)		
	Soy flour/ products	Wheat (semolina)		
		Wheat (white flour)		

SUPER BENEFICIAL	BENEFICIAL	NEUTRAL: Allowed Frequently	NEUTRAL: Allowed Infrequently	AVOID
		100% sprouted grain products (except Essene, Ezekiel)		

Special Variants: *Non-Secretor* NEUTRAL (Allowed Frequently): buckwheat, Ezekiel bread, oat (all), soba noodles (100% buckwheat), soy flour/products, teff; AVOID: cornmeal, couscous, grits, popcorn, wheat (all).

Vegetables

Vegetables provide a rich source of antioxidants and fiber, in addition to helping to lower the production of toxins in the digestive tract. Onions are highly beneficial. They contain significant amounts of the antioxidant quercetin, as well as beneficial polysaccharides, known to aid blood sugar regulation. Many vegetables are rich in potassium, which helps reduce water weight. The common white domestic "silver dollar" mushroom contains diabetes-fighting lectins. Yams are typically high in the amino acid phenylalanine, which inactivates the fat-busting enzyme intestinal alkaline phosphatase (already quite low in Blood Type A), and should be avoided completely.

An item's value also applies to its juice, unless otherwise noted.

BLOOD TYPE A: VEGETABLES			
Portion: 1 cup, prepared (cooked or raw)			
	African	Caucasian	Asian
Secretor	Unlimited	Unlimited	Unlimited
Non-Secretor	Unlimited	Unlimited	Unlimited
		Times per day	

SUPER BENEFICIAL	BENEFICIAL	NEUTRAL: Allowed Frequently	NEUTRAL: Allowed Infrequently	AVOID
Beet greens	Alfalfa sprout	Arugula	Corn	Cabbage
Broccoli	Aloe	Asparagus	Pickle (in brine)	Eggplant
Collard	Artichoke	Asparagus pea	Squash (all)	Mushroom (shiitake)
Dandelion	Bean (green/ snap/ string)	Avocado		Olive (all)
Escarole		Bamboo shoot		Peppers (all)
Mushroom (maitake/ silver dollar)	Carrot	Beet		Pickle (in vinegar)
	Celery	Bok choy		Potato
Onion (all)	Chicory	Brussels sprout		Potato (sweet)
Pea (green/ pod/ snow)	Fennel	Cabbage (juice)*		Rhubarb
Pumpkin	Garlic	Cauliflower		Tomato
Rappini (broccoli rabe)	Horse- radish	Celeriac		Yam
	Kale	Cucumber		Yucca
Spinach	Kohlrabi	Daikon radish		
Swiss chard	Leek	Endive		
	Lettuce (romaine)	Fiddlehead fern		
	Okra	Lettuce (except romaine)		
	Parsnip	Mung bean/ sprouts		
	Turnip	Mushroom (abalone/ enoki/ oyster porto- bello/ straw/ tree ear)		

SUPER BENEFICIAL	BENEFICIAL	NEUTRAL: Allowed Frequently	NEUTRAL: Allowed Infrequently	AVOID
		Mustard greens		
		Oyster plant		
		Poi		
		Radicchio		
		Radish/ sprouts		
		Rutabaga		
		Scallion		
		Seaweed		
		Shallot		
		Taro		
		Water chestnut		
		Watercress		
		Zucchini		

Special Variants: *Non-Secretor* NEUTRAL (Allowed Frequently): alfalfa sprouts, aloe, carrot, celery, eggplant, fennel, garlic, horseradish, lettuce (romaine), mushroom (maitake/shiitake), peppers (all), potato (sweet), rappini, taro, tomato; AVOID: olive, pickles (in brine).

*To obtain the benefits of cabbage juice, it must be consumed within one minute of juicing.

Fruits and Fruit Juices

Fruits are rich in antioxidants and many, such as blueberries, elderberries, cherries, and blackberries, contain polysaccharides that aid weight loss by tempering the effects of insulin. Also, fruits can help shift the balance of water in the body from high extracellular concentrations (edema) to high intracellular concentrations. Many fruits, such as pineapple, are rich in enzymes that can help reduce inflammation and encourage proper water balance. Other fruits, such as red grapefruit and guava, replace tomatoes as rich sources of the antioxidant lycopene. If you have extreme sugar sensitivities, limit your consumption of high-glucose fruits such as grapes and figs.

An item's value also applies to its juice, unless otherwise noted.

BLOOD TYPE A: FRUITS AND FRUIT JUICES			
Portion: 1 cup or 1 piece			
	African	Caucasian	Asian
Secretor	2–4	3–4	3–4
Non-Secretor	2–3	2–3	2–3
		Times per day	

SUPER BENEFICIAL	BENEFICIAL	NEUTRAL: Allowed Frequently	NEUTRAL: Allowed Infrequently	AVOID
Blackberry	Apricot	Apple	Currant	Banana
Blueberry	Boysen-berry	Asian pear	Date	Bitter melon
Cherry	Cranberry	Breadfruit	Grape (all)	Coconut
Pineapple	Elderberry (dark blue/purple)	Canang melon	Pomegran-ate	Honeydew
Plum		Cantaloupe	Quince	Mango
Prune	Fig (fresh/dried)	Casaba melon	Raisin	Orange
	Grapefruit	Christmas melon	Star fruit (caram-bola)	Papaya
	Lemon	Cranberry (juice)	Strawberry	Plantain
	Lime	Crenshaw melon		Tangerine
		Dewberry		
		Gooseberry		
		Guava		
		Kiwi		
		Kumquat		
		Loganberry		
		Mulberry		
		Muskmelon		
		Nectarine		
		Peach		

(handwritten annotations: "CRANBERRY WATERMELON" under Super Beneficial; "BANANA" near Apple; "COCONUT" near Christmas melon; "LIME" and "MANGO" near Loganberry; "CANTALOUPE", "CASABA MELON" near Avoid column)

SUPER BENEFICIAL	BENEFICIAL	NEUTRAL: Allowed Frequently	NEUTRAL: Allowed Infrequently	AVOID
		Pear		
		Persian melon		
		Persimmon		
		PLANTAIN Prickly pear		
		Raspberry		
		Sago palm		
		Spanish melon		
		TANGERINE Watermelon		
		Youngberry		

Special Variants: *Non-Secretor* BENEFICIAL: cranberry (juice), watermelon; NEUTRAL (Allowed Frequently): banana, coconut, lime, mango, plantain, tangerine; AVOID: cantaloupe, casaba melon.

Spices/Condiments/Sweeteners

Many spices have mild to moderate medicinal properties, often by influencing the levels of bacteria in the lower colon. Turmeric contains a powerful phytochemical called curcumin, which helps reduce the levels of intestinal toxins. Baker's and brewer's yeast are beneficial foods for Blood Type A non-secretors, enhancing glucose metabolism and helping ensure a healthy flora balance in the intestinal tract. Many common food additives, such as guar gum and carrageenan, should be avoided, as they can enhance the effects of lectins found in other foods.

SUPER BENEFICIAL	BENEFICIAL	NEUTRAL: Allowed Frequently	NEUTRAL: Allowed Infrequently	AVOID
Fenugreek	Barley malt	Agar	Brown rice syrup	Aspartame
Ginger	Garlic	Allspice	Chocolate	Capers
Turmeric		Almond extract	Cornstarch	Carrageenan

SUPER BENEFICIAL	BENEFICIAL	NEUTRAL: Allowed Frequently	NEUTRAL: Allowed Infrequently	AVOID
	Horserad-ish	Anise	Corn syrup	Chili powder
	Molasses (black-strap)	Apple pectin	Dextrose	Gelatin (except veg-sourced)
	Mustard (dry)	Arrowroot	Fructose	Gums (acacia/ Arabic/ guar)
	Parsley	Basil	Guarana	Juniper
	Soy sauce	Bay leaf	Honey	Ketchup
	Tamari (wheat-free)	Bergamot	Maltodex-trin	Mayonnaise
		Caraway	Maple syrup	MSG
		Cardamom	Rice syrup	Pepper (black/ white)
		Carob	Sugar, (brown/ white)	Pepper (cayenne)
		Chervil		Pepper (pep-percorn/ red flakes
		Chive		Pickles/ relish
		Cilantro (coriander leaf)		Sucanat
		Cinnamon		Vinegar (all)
		Clove		Wintergreen
		Coriander		Worcester-shire sauce
		Cream of tartar		
		Cumin		
		Dill		
		Licorice root*		
		Mace		
		Marjoram		
		Mint (all)		
		Molasses		
		Nutmeg		
		Oregano		
		Paprika		
		Rosemary		
		Saffron		

SUPER BENEFICIAL	BENEFICIAL	NEUTRAL: Allowed Frequently	NEUTRAL: Allowed Infrequently	AVOID
		Sage		
		Savory		
		Sea salt		
		Seaweed		
		Senna		
		Stevia		
		Tamarind		
		Tarragon		
		Thyme		
		Vanilla		
		Vegetable glycerine		
		Yeast (baker's/ brewer's)		

Special Variants: *Non-Secretor* BENEFICIAL: cilantro (coriander leaf), yeast (baker's/ brewer's); NEUTRAL (Allowed Frequently): chili powder, parsley, soy sauce, tamari (wheat-free), turmeric, wintergreen; AVOID: agar, cornstarch, corn syrup, senna.

*Do not use if you have high blood pressure.

Herbal Teas

SUPER BENEFICIAL	BENEFICIAL	NEUTRAL: Allowed Frequently	NEUTRAL: Allowed Infrequently	AVOID
Chamomile	Alfalfa	Chickweed	Hops	Catnip
Dandelion	Aloe	Coltsfoot		Cayenne
Fenugreek	Burdock	Dong Quai		Corn silk
Ginger	Echinacea	Elderberry		Red clover
Ginseng	Gentian	Goldenseal		Rhubarb
Holy basil	Ginkgo biloba	Hore-hound		Yellow dock
	Hawthorn			

SUPER BENEFICIAL	BENEFICIAL	NEUTRAL: Allowed Frequently	NEUTRAL: Allowed Infrequently	AVOID
	Milk thistle	Licorice root*		
	Parsley	Linden		
	Rose hip	Mulberry		
	St. John's wort	Mullein		
	Slippery elm	Peppermint		
	Stone root	Raspberry leaf		
	Valerian	Sage		
		Sarsaparilla		
		Senna		
		Shepherd's purse		
		Skullcap		
		Spearmint		
		Strawberry leaf		
		Thyme		
		White birch		
		White oak bark		
		Yarrow		

Special Variants: *Non-Secretor* AVOID: senna.

*Avoid if you have high blood pressure.

Miscellaneous Beverages

You may wish to have a glass of wine occasionally; you derive substantial benefit to the cardiovascular system from moderate use. Green tea should be part of every Blood Type A health plan. Blood Type As who are not caffeine sensitive might consider having one cup of coffee daily; it contains many enzymes also found in soy that can help your endocrine system function more effectively.

SUPER BENEFICIAL	BENEFICIAL	NEUTRAL: Allowed Frequently	NEUTRAL: Allowed Infrequently	AVOID
Tea (green)	Coffee (regular) Wine (red)	Coffee (decaf) Wine (white)		Beer
				Liquor
				Seltzer
				Soda (club)
				Soda (cola/diet/ misc.)
				Tea, black (reg/ decaf)

Special Variants: *Non-Secretor* BENEFICIAL: wine (white); NEUTRAL (Allowed Frequently): beer, seltzer water, soda (club), tea (black: reg/decaf).

Supplement Protocols

THE DIET FOR BLOOD TYPE A offers abundant quantities of important nutrients. It's vital to get as many nutrients as possible from fresh foods, and to use supplements only to fill in the minor blanks in your diet. The following Supplement Protocols are designed for metabolic enhancement, diabetes management, and support for treatment of diabetic complications. For information about specially formulated, blood type–specific supplements, visit our Web site, www.dadamo.com.

Note: If you are taking insulin or diabetes medications, or are being treated for a related condition, consult your doctor before taking any supplements.

Blood Type A: Pre-Diabetes/ Metabolic Enhancement Protocol

For support of overall metabolic health and blood sugar regulation		
SUPPLEMENT	**ACTION**	**DOSAGE**
High-potency multivitamin, preferably blood type–specific	Nutritional support	As directed
High-potency mineral complex, preferably blood type–specific	Nutritional support	As directed
Larch arabinogalactan	Promotes intestinal health; excellent fiber source	1 tablespoon, twice daily, in juice or water
Probiotic	Promotes intestinal health	1–2 capsules, twice daily
L-carnitine	Promotes metabolic health, energy, active tissue mass	20 mg daily
Holy basil (*Ocimum sanctum*)	Improves stress response	500 mg, 1–2 capsules, twice daily

Blood Type A: Type 1 Diabetes Adjunct

Add these supplements for type 1 diabetes		
SUPPLEMENT	**ACTION**	**DOSAGE**
Quercetin	Prevents diabetic complications	300–600 mg, twice daily
Zinc	Prevents deficiency common to type 1 diabetics	25 mg daily

Blood Type A: Type 2 Diabetes Adjunct

Add these supplements for type 2 diabetes		
SUPPLEMENT	**ACTION**	**DOSAGE**
Quercetin	Prevents diabetic complications	300–600 mg, twice daily
Fenugreek	Lowers blood sugar, improves glucose tolerance	300–600 mg, twice daily
Asian ginseng	Stabilizes blood sugar, prevents post-meal hyperglycemia	100–300 mg, 40 minutes before eating (avoid if you have high blood pressure)

Blood Type A: Diabetic Complications Adjunct

Add these supplements, as appropriate, to support treatment for diabetic complications		
SUPPLEMENT	**ACTION**	**DOSAGE**
Gotu Kola (*Centella asiatica*)	Improves circulation, promotes wound healing, lowers blood pressure	100 mg, 1–2 capsules, twice daily (do not take if you are pregnant)
Vitamin E	Acts as an antioxidant and promotes healing	400 iu daily
Evening primrose oil	Improves nerve function, relieves symptoms of diabetic neuropathy	500 mg, 2 capsules, twice daily
Dandelion (*Taraxacum officinale*)	Reduces edema	250 mg capsule daily, or fresh in salad or tea
Stinging nettle root (*Urtica dioica*)	Reduces edema	500 mg, 1–2 times daily, away from meals

The Exercise Component

FOR BLOOD TYPE A, stress regulation and overall fitness depend on engaging in regular exercises, with an emphasis on calming exercises such as Hatha yoga and T'ai Chi, as well as light aerobic exercise such as walking.

Hatha yoga has become increasingly popular in Western countries as a method for coping with stress, and in my experience it is an excellent form of exercise for Blood Type A. T'ai Chi, a martial art that is basically a form of moving meditation, has also been studied for its antistress effects. T'ai Chi helps reduce stress, lowers blood pressure, and improves mood.

Brisk walking is the ideal aerobic exercise for Blood Type A, especially when done outdoors in a quiet, natural setting. Walking lowers stress levels, and it is considered to be the best form of exercise for diabetes control.

The following constitutes the ideal exercise regimen for Blood Type A:

EXERCISE	DURATION	FREQUENCY
Hatha yoga	40–50 minutes	3–4 x week
Pilates	40–50 minutes	3–4 x week
T'ai Chi	40–50 minutes	3–4 x week
Aerobics (low-impact)	40–50 minutes	2–3 x week
Treadmill	30 minutes	2–3 x week
Weight training (5–10 lb free weights)	15 minutes	2–3 x week
Cycling (recumbent bike)	30 minutes	2–3 x week
Swimming	30 minutes	2–3 x week
Brisk walking	45 minutes	2–3 x week

Getting Started: The First Month

IF YOU ARE NEW to the Blood Type Diet and exercise plan, the following guidelines will introduce you to the Blood Type A regimen over a period of one month. Follow these recommendations as closely as possible, using a journal to record your personal experience with the diet. In addition to measurable factors, such as weight loss, blood sugar regulation, and blood pressure, take the time to note changes in energy levels, sleep patterns, mood, and overall well-being. Over time you'll learn to manage your diet and exercise patterns to achieve the maximum results.

Blood Type A Diabetes Diet Checklist

Avoid meat. Low levels of hydrochloric acid and intestinal alkaline phosphatase make it indigestible for Blood Type A, and can create a range of metabolic problems. ☐

Derive your primary protein from soy products and fresh seafood. Include regular portions of richly oiled cold-water fish. Fish oils can boost your metabolism. ☐

Don't overdo the grains, especially wheat-derived foods. Avoid wheat if you have a weight problem or high blood sugar. ☐

Eat lots of BENEFICIAL fruits and vegetables. ☐

Liberally consume nuts and seeds. Higher quantities of this food group have significant heart health advantages for you. ☐

Limit sugar, caffeine, and alcohol. These are short-term "fixes" that ultimately increase stress and slow down your metabolism. ☐

Don't undereat or skip meals. Use appropriate blood type snacks between meals if you get hungry. Avoid low-calorie diets. Remember, food deprivation is a huge stress. It raises cortisol levels, lowers metabolism, encourages fat storage, and depletes healthy muscle mass. ☐

Eat a balanced breakfast, with more protein-containing food. For Blood Type A, breakfast should be thought of as the "King ☐

of Meals," particularly if you're trying to lose weight. It is the most important meal for balancing your metabolic needs and your stress response.

You'll digest and metabolize foods more efficiently if you avoid eating starches and proteins at the same meal. The use of digestive bitters 30 minutes prior to a meal can also help you digest foods more efficiently. ☐

Week 1

Blood Type Diet and Supplements

- Cut back or eliminate your most harmful AVOID foods—red meat, the majority of noncultured dairy foods, and beans that have an insulinlike effect for your blood type, such as lima, kidney, and navy beans. These foods seriously interfere with proper metabolism.
- If you are a non-secretor, cut down on or eliminate wheat.
- Include your most important BENEFICIAL foods at least five times this week.
- Incorporate at least two or three SUPER BENEFICIAL foods into your daily diet. For example, have a handful of peanuts as a snack, toss some fresh blueberries into your morning cereal, have a glass of soy milk in midafternoon.
- While it's okay for you to have a cup of coffee every day if you're not caffeine-sensitive, make sure to drink at least one or two cups of SUPER BENEFICIAL green tea every day (my favorite is Itaru's Premium Green Tea, which you can order from our Web site).
- To improve blood sugar regulation, eat 5 to 6 small meals throughout the day, rather than 3 large meals.

Exercise Regimen

- Plan to exercise at least 4 days this week, for 45 minutes each day.
  2 days: walking or light aerobic activity
  2 days: yoga or T'ai Chi
- Use your journal to detail the time, activity, distance, and amount of weight. Note the repetitions used for each exercise.

Start slowly, giving yourself a chance to get used to the Blood Type A Diet. You'll have a much better chance of long-term success if you take some time to incorporate the Blood Type Diet recommendations into your daily life. I've found that the biggest indicator of failure is a rigid adherence to the plan from the first day on. I know you want to get moving and start seeing results. That's a positive goal. But patience is your friend if you want to make a permanent change in your diet and lifestyle.

Week 2

Blood Type Diet and Supplements

- Begin to eliminate the next level of AVOID foods—potatoes, beans, and legumes.
- Eat at least two to three BENEFICIAL proteins every day, favoring seafood, soy, and cultured dairy.
- Continue to incorporate SUPER BENEFICIAL foods into your daily diet.
- Continue to eat 5 to 6 small meals throughout the day, rather than 3 large meals.
- Choose the NEUTRAL foods listed as "Allowed Frequently" over those listed as "Allowed Infrequently."

Exercise Regimen

- Continue to exercise at least 4 days this week, for 45 minutes each day.
  2 days: walking or light aerobic activity
  2 days: yoga or T'ai Chi
- Take a couple of relaxation breaks during the workday, especially if you have a high-stress job, or one that requires great concentration. Close your office door, turn off the light, and do some deep breathing and relaxation exercises. You will return to work after twenty minutes refreshed and more alert.

Don't leave home without a quick energy snack tucked into your purse or briefcase.

- Super Smoothie in a Thermos, made with 1 tablespoon soy-based protein powder, blended with 2 cups berries and ½ cup pineapple juice
- Trail mix: peanuts, walnuts, pumpkin seeds, dried pineapple

Week 3

Blood Type Diet and Supplements

- When you plan your meals for week 3, choose BENEFICIAL foods to replace NEUTRAL foods whenever possible. For example, choose tofu over chicken, or a plum instead of an apple.
- Eliminate all remaining AVOID foods.
- Liberally incorporate SUPER BENEFICIAL foods into your daily diet.
- Continue to eat 5 to 6 small meals throughout the day, rather than 3 large meals.

Exercise Regimen

- Continue to exercise at least 4 days this week, for 45 minutes each day.
  2 days: walking or light aerobic activity
  2 days: yoga or T'ai Chi
- Add one day of unstructured exercise—walking, biking, swimming.

■ WEEK 3 SUCCESS STRATEGY ■

Make your meals times of relaxation, not anxiety. Always eat sitting down, avoid stressful discussions, and chew each bite slowly, putting down your fork between bites.

Week 4

Blood Type Diet

- Continue at the week 3 level, focusing on BENEFICIAL and SUPER BENEFICIAL foods.
- Continue to eat 5 to 6 small meals throughout the day, rather than 3 large meals.

- If you haven't already done so, find out your secretor status. (See Appendix B to order the test.) If you're a non-secretor, increase your compliance by making the recommended adjustments in your diet.

Exercise Regimen

- Continue at the week 3 level.

- Evaluate your progress, referring to your journal. Determine which exercise regimen has worked for you, including time of day, setting, and activity level. Look for ways to improve your performance and endurance.

■ WEEK 4 SUCCESS STRATEGY ■

If you are experiencing anxiety or sleep deprivation, I recommend a technique called alternate nostril breathing. Left nostril breathing generates a more relaxing effect. Right nostril breathing generates a more energized effect. Switching back and forth tends to balance your nervous system. Holding your right nostril closed, breathe slowly through the left nostril to the count of ten. Switch nostrils and repeat. Perform the exercise five times.

FAQs: Blood Type A and Diabetes

I have constant sugar cravings, even when I stick closely to the diet for Blood Type A. Any suggestions?

Very often, this type of sugar reaction complicates an otherwise nice result from the diet. Usually it is just that the liver is having some problems adjusting to the new way of eating and needs some rehabilitation. Try taking the herb milk thistle for a few weeks, and drink a cup of licorice root tea at about 10:00 A.M. and 2:00 P.M. (Do not use licorice without your doctor's approval if you suffer from high blood pressure. DGL—deglycyrrhyzinated licorice—is preferable for you.)

I've cut down on cigarettes and now smoke less than ten a day— down from two packs. I am concerned about gaining weight and making my blood sugar problems worse if I quit altogether.

There are many reasons to quit smoking, especially for Blood Type A, who is most vulnerable to all smoking-related diseases. To address your concern, if you smoke because you fear the weight gain that might come with quitting, consider this: Cigarette smokers tend to be more insulin-resistant, compared with nonsmokers. In effect, smoking is bound to create the very condition you fear.

Won't eating wheat slow down my metabolism?

If you are a Blood Type A non-secretor, you have a greater sensitivity to complex carbohydrates, especially wheat, whose lectins can exert an insulinlike effect—lowering active tissue mass and increasing total body fat. I would recommend that non-secretors strictly limit or avoid wheat. Even Blood Type A secretors should use moderation in the consumption of wheat if they are diabetic.

I've read that lycopene is a beneficial nutrient contained in tomatoes. Since Blood Type A must avoid tomatoes, is there another way to get lycopene?

Replace tomatoes with a Membrane Fluidizer Cocktail, designed for Blood Type A. Using guava, ruby red grapefruit, or watermelon juice as the base, add 1/2 to 1 tablespoon of high-quality flaxseed oil and 1 tablespoon of good-quality lecithin. Shake well. The lecithin emulsifies the oil, giving the drink a "smoothie" texture. This formulation increases the absorption of lycopene from these foods to the level of tomato paste, but without the tomato lectin.

I am a postmenopausal diabetic woman. I am concerned about not getting enough calcium in my diet, since most meat and dairy foods are AVOIDs for Blood Type A.

Postmenopausal women who are Blood Type A have special challenges when it comes to getting enough calcium and absorbing it properly. You have low levels of intestinal alkaline phosphatase and stomach acid, factors known to impair calcium metabolism. You can increase your consumption of calcium and its absorption in the following ways:

1. Regularly consume low-fat yogurt, soy milk, and goat milk.
2. Include lots of almonds, broccoli, and dark leafy greens like chards, collards, kale, and spinach in your diet.

3. Take a daily dose of supplemental calcium citrate—300 to 600 mg.
4. Follow the exercise regimen for Blood Type A, and do as much walking as you can.

A Final Word

IN SUMMARY, the secret to fighting diabetes with the Blood Type A Diet involves:

1. Increasing active tissue mass (calorie-burning tissue) by eating a diet rich in soy protein, healthy seafood, and green vegetables.
2. Minimizing consumption of the insulin-mimicking lectins, abundant in AVOID beans, grains, and vegetables that are not recommended for your blood type.
3. Improving your metabolic health, lowering your cholesterol, controlling your blood pressure, and lowering your risk for heart disease by avoiding red meat and high-fat foods.
4. Reducing cortisol levels by engaging in regular exercise—and by not overdoing it.
5. Using supplements intelligently to block the effect of insulin-mimicking lectins, provide antioxidant support, and protect delicate nerve tissue from destruction.

SIX

Blood Type

B

THE PRIMARY CHALLENGE FACED BY BLOOD TYPE B IN MAIN-taining a healthy weight, regulating blood sugar, and achieving metabolic balance is a sensitivity to B-specific lectins in select foods. Secondary factors contributing to metabolic imbalance include the consumption of foods containing opposing antigens (for example, A-like), and the colonization of the gut by anti-B bacteria. These factors can contribute to insulin resistance and heighten your risk for developing Metabolic Syndrome. Lectins can cause insulin resistance, resulting in weight gain, fluid retention, and hypoglycemia. When food is not efficiently digested and burned as fuel for the body, it gets stored as fat.

If you are a non-secretor, you have a greater susceptibility to Metabolic Syndrome, which can cause impairment of triglyceride conversion, resulting in elevated blood lipid levels and a slowed metabolic rate. Sluggish metabolism also promotes the storage of excess fluid as extracellular water.

Since dairy foods are encouraged in the Blood Type B Diet, some of my Type B patients worry about gaining weight. It's certainly true that if you overeat high-fat, high-calorie dairy foods, you'll probably gain weight. However, the moderate consumption of dairy foods, particularly cultured products like kefir and yogurt, aids your digestion, promotes healthy bowel flora, and increases active tissue mass. Dairy, used wisely, is good for you.

In addition, idiosyncratic ethnic and racial variations require mixed strategies. It has consistently been my experience that Blood Type Bs of African ancestry initially encounter problems on the diet. African Americans, especially those who are Rh-negative, also appear to have more chronic health problems and are known to produce more anti–blood type antibodies than other Blood Type B individuals. I suspect the basis might be anthropological, since the gene for Blood Type B was extremely rare among the African peoples—awaiting migration to far different altitudes and climatic regions and a long evolutionary process for its full flourishing.

Blood Type B Weight Profile

Weight Gain		Weight Loss	
FOOD	**MECHANISM**	**FOOD**	**MECHANISM**
Chicken	Promotes insulin resistance	Meat, liver	Optimize metabolism and aid digestion
Lentils, peanuts, sesame seeds	Promote insulin resistance/ hypoglycemia	Low-fat dairy	Improves insulin metabolism
Corn, potatoes	Promote insulin resistance	Broccoli, greens	Aid efficient metabolism
Wheat, buckwheat	Promote insulin resistance and impair calorie utilization	Walnuts	Improve insulin production
Processed sugar	Promotes insulin resistance	Licorice tea	Counters hypoglycemia

Since dairy foods are so beneficial for Blood Type B individuals, their absence in the typical African American diet may contribute to some of the additional health problems African Americans face. If you are of African ancestry and are lactose-intolerant, you'll need to introduce dairy foods very gradually. The use of a "lactase" (lactose-digestive enzyme) product can be of great assistance to you in this adjustment phase.

The Diabetes-Stress Factor

BLOOD TYPE Bs who struggle with low metabolism and weight gain have another challenge—the effects of high levels of the stress hormone cortisol. As we described earlier, cortisol promotes insulin resistance and hormonal imbalance.

With Blood Type B's added difficulties due to the stress-cortisol connection, you may need to work a bit harder to stay energized. Try to establish a regular sleep schedule and adhere to it as closely as possible. A normal sleep-wake rhythm is crucial for optimal cortisol release throughout the day. Schedule at least two breaks of twenty minutes each for complete relaxation. Combat sleep disturbances with regular exercise and a relaxing pre-bedtime routine. A light snack before bedtime will help raise your blood sugar levels and improve sleep. Most important, be attentive to the factors in your daily life that elevate your stress levels. When you take steps to eliminate stressors, you are doing more than simply improving your mood. You're protecting your health.

Blood Type B: The Foods

THE BLOOD TYPE B Diabetes Diet is specifically adapted for the prevention and management of diabetes. The new category, **Super Beneficial**, highlights powerful diabetes-fighting foods for Type B. The **Neutral** category has also been adjusted to de-emphasize foods that can cause problems for diabetics. Foods designated **Neutral: Allowed Infrequently** should be minimized or avoided, depending on your condition. Eat these foods no more than once or twice a month.

Food Values

SUPER BENEFICIAL	Foods that are known to have specific disease-fighting qualities for your blood type.
BENEFICIAL	Foods with components that enhance the metabolic, immune, or structural health of your blood type.
NEUTRAL: Allowed Frequently	Foods that normally have no direct blood type effect but supply a variety of nutrients necessary for a healthful diet.
NEUTRAL: Allowed Infrequently	Foods that normally have no blood type effect but may impede your progress when consumed regularly.
AVOID	Foods with components that are harmful to your blood type.

Your secretor status can influence your ability to fully digest and metabolize certain foods, so various adjustments in the values are made for non-secretors. If you do not know your secretor type, the odds are that you can safely use the standard values, since the majority of the population (80 percent) are secretors. However, I urge you to get tested, since the variations are important for non-secretors who want to maximize the effectivenesss of the Blood Type Diet.

The food charts are divided into three sections. The top of the chart suggests the average portion size and quantity per week or day, according to secretor status. These recommendations do *not* apply to the category **Neutral: Allowed Infrequently;** those foods should be consumed sparingly (0–2 times a month). The charts also indicate differences in frequency for some foods, based on ethnic heritage. It has been my experience that this factor has an impact on the individual's ability to fully digest certain foods. For the purposes of blood type food choices, persons of Hispanic heritage should follow the diet recommendations for Caucasians, and North American Native peoples should follow the diet recommendations for Asians.

The middle section of the chart provides the food values. The bottom section lists variants based on secretor status or other key factors.

For your convenience, we have included a number of product names, such as ketchup, Worcestershire sauce, and Ezekiel bread. However, bear in mind that commercial formulations vary among brands and regions. Even though a product may be listed as okay for you, always check its ingredients; do not use products that contain **Avoid** ingredients for your blood type. Of course, you may choose to make your own version of commercial products such as bread and mayonnaise, using ingredients that suit your blood type. There are hundreds of delicious recipes for every blood type available on our Web site (www.dadamo.com) and in the book *Cook Right 4 Your Type: The Practical Kitchen Companion to* Eat Right 4 Your Type.

Meat/Poultry

Blood Type B is able to efficiently metabolize animal protein, but there are some unexpected limitations that require careful dietary navigation. Chicken, one of the most popular food choices, disagrees with Blood Type B because of the lectin contained in the organ and muscle meat. Turkey does not contain this lectin and is an excellent alternative to chicken. The leaner cuts of lamb and mutton should be a part of your diet. They help build muscle and active tissue mass, increasing your metabolic rate. Blood Type B non-secretors require a larger weekly intake of meat and poultry. Choose only the best-quality (preferably grass-fed), antibiotic-, chemical-, and pesticide-free, low-fat meats and poultry.

BLOOD TYPE B: MEATS/POULTRY			
Portion: 4–6 oz (men); 2–5 oz (women and children)			
	African	Caucasian	Asian
Secretor	3–6	2–6	2–5
Non-Secretor	4–7	4–7	4–7
	Times per week		

SUPER BENEFICIAL	BENEFICIAL	NEUTRAL: Allowed Frequently	NEUTRAL: Allowed Infrequently	AVOID
Lamb Mutton	Goat Rabbit Venison	Beef Buffalo Liver (calf) Ostrich Pheasant Turkey Veal		All commercially processed meats Bacon/Ham/Pork Chicken Cornish hen Duck Goose Grouse Guinea hen Heart (beef) Horse Partridge Quail Squab Squirrel Sweetbreads Turtle

Special Variants: *Non-Secretor* BENEFICIAL: liver (calf); NEUTRAL (Allowed Frequently): heart, horse, squab, sweetbreads.

Fish/Seafood

Fish and seafood are an excellent source of protein for Blood Type B. Fish is a treasure trove of dense nutrients and a great builder of active tissue mass, particularly for non-secretors. Seafood is also a good source of docosahexaenoic acid (DHA), a nutrient needed for proper nerve, tissue, and growth function. Many of the AVOID seafoods have lectins that react adversely with Type B blood.

BLOOD TYPE B: FISH/SEAFOOD

Portion: 4–6 oz (men); 2–5 oz (women and children)

	African	Caucasian	Asian
Secretor	4–5	3–5	3–5
Non-Secretor	4–5	4–5	4–5
	Times per week		

SUPER BENEFICIAL	BENEFICIAL	NEUTRAL: Allowed Frequently	NEUTRAL: Allowed Infrequently	AVOID
Cod	Caviar	Abalone	Herring	Anchovy
Halibut	(sturgeon)	Bluefish	(pickled/	Barracuda
Mackerel	Croaker	Bullhead	smoked)	Bass (all)
Sardine	Flounder	Carp	Salmon	Beluga
	Grouper	Catfish	(smoked)	Butterfish
	Haddock	Chub	Scallop	Clam
	Hake	Cusk		Conch
	Harvest fish	Drum		Crab
	Mahi-mahi	Gray sole		Crayfish
	Monkfish	Halfmoon fish		Eel
	Perch (ocean)	Herring (fresh)		Frog
	Pickerel	Mullet		Lobster
	Pike	Muskellunge		Mussels
	Porgy	Opaleye		Octopus
	Salmon	Orange roughy		Oysters
	Shad	Parrot fish		Pollock
	Sole	Perch (silver/white/yellow)		Shrimp
	Sturgeon	Pompano		Snail (Helix pomatia/escargot)
		Red snapper		Trout (all)
				Yellowtail

SUPER BENEFICIAL	BENEFICIAL	NEUTRAL: Allowed Frequently	NEUTRAL: Allowed Infrequently	AVOID
		Rosefish		
		Sailfish		
		Scrod		
		Scup		
		Shark		
		Smelt		
		Sole (all)		
		Squid (calamari)		
		Sucker		
		Sunfish		
		Swordfish		
		Tilapia		
		Tilefish		
		Tuna		
		Weakfish		
		Whitefish		
		Whiting		

Special Variants: *Non-Secretor* BENEFICIAL: carp; NEUTRAL (Allowed Frequently): barracuda, butterfish, caviar (sturgeon), flounder, gray sole, halibut, pike, salmon, snail (*Helix pomatia*), sole, yellowtail; AVOID: scallops.

Dairy/Eggs

Dairy products can be eaten by almost all Blood Type B secretors, and to a lesser degree by non-secretors. Blood Type B can make smart dairy choices to build active tissue mass and increase metabolism. However, non-secretors should be wary of eating too much cheese, as you are more sensitive to many of the microbial strains in aged cheeses. This is more common if you are of African ancestry, but the sensitivity can also be found in Caucasian and Asian populations. Use caution if you suffer from recurrent sinus infections or colds, as dairy products are often mucus producers. Eggs are a good source of DHA for Blood Type B and can be an integral part of your protein requirement, helping to build active tissue mass. Try to find eggs and dairy products that meet organic standards.

BLOOD TYPE B: EGGS			
Portion: 1 egg			
	African	Caucasian	Asian
Secretor	3–4	3–4	3–4
Non-Secretor	5–6	5–6	5–6
		Times per week	

BLOOD TYPE B: MILK AND YOGURT			
Portion: 4–6 oz (men); 2–5 oz (women and children)			
	African	Caucasian	Asian
Secretor	3–5	3–4	3–4
Non-Secretor	1–3	2–4	1–3
		Times per week	

BLOOD TYPE B: CHEESE			
Portion: 3 oz (men); 2 oz (women and children)			
	African	Caucasian	Asian
Secretor	3–4	3–5	3–4
Non-Secretor	1–4	1–4	1–4
		Times per week	

SUPER BENEFICIAL	BENEFICIAL	NEUTRAL: Allowed Frequently	NEUTRAL: Allowed Infrequently	AVOID
Kefir	Cottage	Camem-	Brie	American
Yogurt	cheese	bert	Butter	cheese
	Farmer	Casein	Butter-	Blue cheese
	cheese	Cream	milk	Egg (duck/
	Feta	cheese	Cheddar	goose/
	Goat	Edam	Colby	quail)
	cheese	Egg	Half-and-	Ice cream
	Milk (cow/	(chicken)	half	
	goat)	Emmenthal	Jarlsberg	

SUPER BENEFICIAL	BENEFICIAL	NEUTRAL: Allowed Frequently	NEUTRAL: Allowed Infrequently	AVOID
	Mozzarella Paneer Ricotta	Ghee (clarified butter) Gouda Gruyère Neufchâtel Parmesan Provolone Quark Sour cream	Monterey Jack Muenster Sherbet Swiss cheese Whey	

Special Variants: *Non-Secretor* BENEFICIAL: whey; NEUTRAL (Allowed Frequently): cottage cheese, milk (cow); AVOID: Camembert, cheddar, Emmenthal, Jarlsberg, Monterey Jack, Muenster, Parmesan, provolone, Swiss cheese.

Oils

Blood Type B does best on monounsaturated oils, such as olive oil, and oils rich in omega series fatty acids, such as flaxseed oil. Make it a point to avoid sesame, sunflower, and corn oils, which contain lectins that impair Blood Type B digestion.

BLOOD TYPE B: OILS			
Portion: 1 tblsp			
	African	Caucasian	Asian
Secretor	5–8	5–8	5–8
Non-Secretor	3–7	3–7	3–7
		Times per week	

SUPER BENEFICIAL	BENEFICIAL	NEUTRAL: Allowed Frequently	NEUTRAL: Allowed Infrequently	AVOID
	Olive	Almond Black currant seed Cod liver Evening primrose Flax (linseed) Walnut	Wheat germ	Borage seed Canola Castor Coconut Corn Cottonseed Peanut Safflower Sesame Soy Sunflower
Special Variants: *Non-Secretor* BENEFICIAL: black currant seed, flax (linseed), walnut.				

Nuts and Seeds

Nuts and seeds can be an important secondary source of protein for Blood Type B. In particular, black walnuts can aid bowel health and have properties known to improve blood sugar regulation. As with other aspects of the Blood Type B Diet Plan, there are some idiosyncratic elements to the choice of seeds and nuts. Several, such as sunflower and sesame, have B-agglutinating lectins and should be avoided.

BLOOD TYPE B: NUTS AND SEEDS			
Portion: Whole (handful); Nut Butters (2 tblsp)			
	African	Caucasian	Asian
Secretor	4–7	4–7	4–7
Non-Secretor	5–7	5–7	5–7
		Times per week	

SUPER BENEFICIAL	BENEFICIAL	NEUTRAL: Allowed Frequently	NEUTRAL: Allowed Infrequently	AVOID
Walnut (black)		Almond	Litchi	Cashew
		Almond butter	Macadamia	Filbert (hazelnut)
		Beechnut	Pecan	Peanut
		Brazil nut		Peanut butter
		Butternut		Pignolia (pine nut)
		Chestnut		Pistachio
		Flax (linseed)		Poppy seed
		Hickory		Pumpkin seed
		Walnut (English)		Safflower seed
				Sesame butter (tahini)
				Sesame seed
				Sunflower butter
				Sunflower seed

Special Variants: *Non-Secretor* BENEFICIAL: walnut (English); NEUTRAL (Allowed Frequently): pumpkin seed.

Beans and Legumes

Blood Type B can do well on the proteins found in many beans and legumes, although this food category does contain more than a few beans with problematic lectins. Soy products should be de-emphasized, as they are rich in a class of enzymes that can interact negatively with the B antigen. Several beans, such as mung beans, contain Blood Type B agglutinating lectins and should be avoided.

BLOOD TYPE B: BEANS AND LEGUMES			
Portion: 1 cup (cooked)			
	African	**Caucasian**	**Asian**
Secretor	5–7	5–7	5–7
Non-Secretor	3–5	3–5	3–5
		Times per week	

SUPER BENEFICIAL	BENEFICIAL	NEUTRAL: Allowed Frequently	NEUTRAL: Allowed Infrequently	AVOID
Bean (green/ snap/ string)	Kidney bean	Cannellini bean		Adzuki bean
	Lima bean	Copper bean		Black bean
Fava (broad) bean	Navy bean	Jicama bean		Black-eyed pea
Northern bean		Pea (green/ pod/ snow)		Garbanzo (chickpea)
		Tamarind bean		Lentil (all)
		White bean		Miso
				Mung bean/ sprouts
				Pinto bean
				Soy bean
				Soy cheese
				Soy milk
				Tempeh
				Tofu

Special Variants: *Non-Secretor* NEUTRAL (Allowed Frequently): bean (green/snap/ string), fava (broad) bean, kidney bean, lima bean, navy bean, northern bean, soy milk.

Grains and Starches

Grains present a series of problems for Blood Type B, especially in the area of insulin regulation. Non-secretors should be even more circum-spect about consumption of complex carbohydrates because of their somewhat less stable insulin response. Corn lectin increases body fat for Blood Type B, as do corn by-products. Rye and buckwheat should also be avoided; these foods contain lectins capable of exerting an insulinlike effect on your body, resulting in a decrease of active tissue mass and an increase in body fat. Minimize or avoid whole-wheat products. The agglutinin in whole wheat can aggravate inflammatory conditions and lower active tissue mass. This lectin can often be milled out of the grain or destroyed by sprouting.

BLOOD TYPE B: GRAINS AND STARCHES			
Portion: 1 cup dry (grains or pastas); 1 muffin; 2 slices of bread			
	African	Caucasian	Asian
Secretor	5–7	5–9	5–9
Non-Secretor	3–5	3–5	3–5
			Times per week

SUPER BENEFICIAL	BENEFICIAL	NEUTRAL: Allowed Frequently	NEUTRAL: Allowed Infrequently	AVOID
	Essene bread (Manna)	Barley	Rice (white/ brown/ basmati)	Amaranth
	Millet	Ezekiel 4:9 bread	Rice flour	Barley
	Oat bran	Quinoa	Soy flour/ products	Buckwheat
	Oat flour	Spelt flour/ products	Wheat (re-fined, un-bleached)	Cornmeal
	Oatmeal		Wheat (semolina)	Couscous
	Rice bran		Wheat (white flour)	Kamut
	Rice cake			Popcorn
	Rice milk			Rice (wild)
	Spelt (whole)			Rye
				Rye flour
				Soba noodles (100% buck-wheat)
				Sorghum

SUPER BENEFICIAL	BENEFICIAL	NEUTRAL: Allowed Frequently	NEUTRAL: Allowed Infrequently	AVOID
				Tapioca
				Teff
				Wheat (whole)
				Wheat bran
				Wheat germ

Special Variants: *Non-Secretor* NEUTRAL (Allowed Frequently): amaranth, oat (all), rice (wild), sorghum, spelt (whole), tapioca; AVOID: soy flour/products, wheat (all).

Vegetables

Vegetables provide a rich source of antioxidants and fiber and also help to lower the production of toxins in the digestive tract. Many vegetables are rich in potassium, which helps to lower extracellular water (edema) in the body while raising the levels of intracellular water. All of the beneficial vegetables are effective for Blood Type Bs, particularly if you are trying to lose weight. Mushrooms are great for Blood Type B diabetics. Research shows that the mushroom lectin (*Agaricus bisporus*) stimulates insulin release from the pancreas and aids proper insulin regulation.

An item's value also applies to its juice, unless otherwise noted.

BLOOD TYPE B: VEGETABLES			
Portion: 1 cup, prepared (cooked or raw)			
	African	Caucasian	Asian
Secretor	Unlimited	Unlimited	Unlimited
Non-Secretor	Unlimited	Unlimited	Unlimited
	Times per day		

SUPER BENEFICIAL	BENEFICIAL	NEUTRAL: Allowed Frequently	NEUTRAL: Allowed Infrequently	AVOID
Beet	Brussels sprout	Alfalfa sprouts	Potato	Aloe
Beet greens	Cabbage*	Arugula		Artichoke
Broccoli	Carrot	Asparagus		Corn
Collard	Cauli-flower	Asparagus pea		Olive (all)
Kale	Eggplant	Bamboo shoot		Pumpkin
Mushroom (shiitake)	Parsnip	Bean (green/ snap/ string)		Radish/ sprouts
Mustard greens	Peppers (all)	Bok choy		Rhubarb
	Potato (sweet)	Carrot (juice)		Tomato
	Yam	Celeriac		
		Celery		
		Chicory		
		Cucumber		
		Daikon radish		
		Dandelion		
		Endive		
		Escarole		
		Fennel		
		Fiddlehead fern		
		Garlic		
		Horse-radish		
		Kohlrabi		
		Leek		
		Lettuce (all)		

SUPER BENEFICIAL	BENEFICIAL	NEUTRAL: Allowed Frequently	NEUTRAL: Allowed Infrequently	AVOID
		Mushroom (abalone/ enoki/ maitake/ oyster/ porto- bello/ silver dollar/ straw/ tree ear)		
		Okra		
		Onion (all)		
		Oyster plant		
		Pea (green/ pod/snow)		
		Pickle (in brine or vinegar)		
		Poi		
		Radicchio		
		Rappini (broccoli rabe)		
		Rutabaga		
		Scallion		
		Seaweed		
		Shallot		
		Spinach		
		Squash (all)		
		Swiss chard		
		Taro		
		Turnip		
		Water chestnut		
		Watercress		

SUPER BENEFICIAL	BENEFICIAL	NEUTRAL: Allowed Frequently	NEUTRAL: Allowed Infrequently	AVOID
		Yucca Zucchini		

Special Variants: *Non-Secretor* BENEFICIAL: garlic, okra, onion (all); NEUTRAL (Allowed Frequently): artichoke, cabbage, eggplant, peppers (all), pumpkin, tomato; AVOID: potato.

*To obtain the benefits of cabbage juice, it must be consumed within one minute of juicing.

Fruits and Fruit Juices

Fruits are a terrific source of antioxidants. Blueberries, elderberries, cherries, and blackberries contain polysaccharides that block the liver enzyme ornithine decarboxylase (ODC). This has the effect of lowering the production of toxic chemicals (polyamines) in the intestinal tract. A diet rich in proper fruits and vegetables can encourage weight loss by tempering the effects of insulin. Also, fruits can help shift the balance of water in the body from high extracellular concentrations (edema) to high intracellular concentrations. Pineapples are rich in enzymes that help reduce inflammation and encourage proper water balance.

An item's value also applies to its juice, unless otherwise noted.

BLOOD TYPE B: FRUITS AND FRUIT JUICES			
Portion: 1 cup			
	African	Caucasian	Asian
Secretor	2–4	3–5	3–5
Non-Secretor	2–3	2–3	2–3
	Times per day		

SUPER BENEFICIAL	BENEFICIAL	NEUTRAL: Allowed Frequently	NEUTRAL: Allowed Infrequently	AVOID
Cranberry	Banana	Apple	Apricot	Avocado
Elderberry	Grape	Blackberry	Asian pear	Bitter melon
Pineapple	Papaya	Blueberry		Coconut

SUPER BENEFICIAL	BENEFICIAL	NEUTRAL: Allowed Frequently	NEUTRAL: Allowed Infrequently	AVOID
Water-melon	Plum	Boysen-berry	Breadfruit	Persimmon
		Canang melon	Cantaloupe	Pomegranate
		Casaba melon	Currant	Prickly pear
		Cherry (all)	Date	Star fruit (carambola)
		Christmas melon	Fig (fresh/dried)	
		Crenshaw melon	Honeydew melon	
		Dewberry	Plantain	
		Gooseberry	Raisin	
		Grapefruit		
		Guava		
		Kiwi		
		Kumquat		
		Lemon		
		Lime		
		Loganberry		
		Mango		
		Mulberry		
		Muskmelon		
		Nectarine		
		Orange		
		Peach		
		Pear		
		Persian melon		
		Prune		
		Quince		
		Raspberry		
		Sago palm		

SUPER BENEFICIAL	BENEFICIAL	NEUTRAL: Allowed Frequently	NEUTRAL: Allowed Infrequently	AVOID
		Spanish melon Strawberry Tangerine Young-berry		

Special Variants: *Non-Secretor* BENEFICIAL: blackberry, blueberry, boysenberry, cherry, currant, elderberry, fig (dried/fresh), guava, raspberry; NEUTRAL (Allowed Frequently): banana; AVOID: cantaloupe, honeydew.

Spices/Condiments/Sweeteners

Many spices have mild to moderate medicinal properties. Some exert a beneficial influence on the bacterial balance in the lower intestine. Many common food additives, such as guar gum and carrageenan, should be avoided. They can enhance the effects of lectins found in other foods. Brewer's yeast is a beneficial food for Blood Type B non-secretors. It enhances glucose metabolism and helps ensure a healthy flora balance in the intestinal tract. Type B responds best to warming herbs, such as ginger, horseradish, and cayenne pepper.

SUPER BENEFICIAL	BENEFICIAL	NEUTRAL: Allowed Frequently	NEUTRAL: Allowed Infrequently	AVOID
Fenugreek Ginger	Horserad-ish Molasses (black-strap) Parsley Pepper (cayenne)	Anise Apple pectin Basil Bay leaf Bergamot Caper Caraway Cardamom	Agar Arrowroot Chocolate Fructose Honey Maple syrup Mayon-naise	Allspice Almond extract Aspartame Barley malt Carrageenan Cinnamon Cornstarch Corn syrup

SUPER BENEFICIAL	BENEFICIAL	NEUTRAL: Allowed Frequently	NEUTRAL: Allowed Infrequently	AVOID
		Carob	Molasses	Dextrose
		Chervil	Pickles (all)	Gelatin (except veg-sourced)
		Chili powder	Rice syrup	
		Chive	Sugar (brown/white)	Guarana
		Cilantro (coriander leaf)	Tamari (wheat-free)	Gums (acacia/Arabic/guar)
		Clove	Vinegar (all)	Juniper
		Coriander		Ketchup
		Cream of tartar		Malto-dextrin
		Cumin		Miso
		Dill		MSG
		Garlic		Pepper (black/white)
		Lecithin		Soy sauce
		Mace		Stevia
		Marjoram		Sucanat
		Mint (all)		Tapioca
		Mustard (dry)		
		Nutmeg		
		Oregano		
		Paprika		
		Pepper (peppercorn/red flakes)		
		Rosemary		
		Saffron		
		Sage		
		Savory		
		Sea salt		
		Seaweed		

SUPER BENEFICIAL	BENEFICIAL	NEUTRAL: Allowed Frequently	NEUTRAL: Allowed Infrequently	AVOID
		Senna		
		Tamarind		
		Tarragon		
		Thyme		
		Turmeric		
		Vanilla		
		Wintergreen		
		Yeast (baker's/ brewer's)		

Special Variants: *Non-Secretor* BENEFICIAL: brewer's yeast, oregano; NEUTRAL (Allowed Frequently): stevia; AVOID: agar, fructose, pickle relish, sugar (brown/white).

Herbal Teas

SUPER BENEFICIAL	BENEFICIAL	NEUTRAL: Allowed Frequently	NEUTRAL: Allowed Infrequently	AVOID
Dandelion	Ginseng	Alfalfa	Dong Quai	Aloe
Ginger	Parsley	Burdock		Coltsfoot
Licorice root*	Pepper-mint	Catnip		Corn silk
	Raspberry leaf	Chamomile		Fenugreek
	Rosehip	Chickweed		Gentian
	Sage	Echinacea		Hops
		Elder		Linden
		Goldenseal		Mullein
		Hawthorn		Red clover
		Horehound		Rhubarb
		Mulberry		Shepherd's purse
		Rosemary		Skullcap
		Sarsaparilla		
		Senna		

*Avoid if you have high blood pressure.

SUPER BENEFICIAL	BENEFICIAL	NEUTRAL: Allowed Frequently	NEUTRAL: Allowed Infrequently	AVOID
		Slippery elm		
		Spearmint		
		St. John's wort		
		Strawberry leaf		
		Thyme		
		Valerian		
		Vervain		
		White birch		
		White oak bark		
		Yarrow		
		Yellow dock		

Miscellaneous Beverages

Blood Type B non-secretors may wish to have a glass of wine occasionally. There are substantial cardiovascular benefits from moderate use. Green tea is an excellent substitute for coffee.

SUPER BENEFICIAL	BENEFICIAL	NEUTRAL: Allowed Frequently	NEUTRAL: Allowed Infrequently	AVOID
Tea (green)		Wine (red/ white)	Beer	Liquor
			Coffee (reg/ decaf)	Seltzer
				Soda (club)
			Tea, black (reg/ decaf)	Soda (cola/ diet/misc.)

Special Variants: *Non-Secretor* BENEFICIAL: wine (red/white); NEUTRAL (Allowed Frequently): liquor, seltzer, soda (club); AVOID: coffee (reg/decaf), tea (black, reg/decaf).

Supplement Protocols

THE DIET FOR BLOOD TYPE B offers abundant quantities of important nutrients. It's vital to get as many nutrients as possible from fresh foods and to use supplements only to fill in the minor blanks in your diet. The following Supplement Protocols are designed for metabolic enhancement, diabetes management, and support for treatment of diabetic complications. For information about specially formulated blood type–specific supplements, visit our Web site, www.dadamo.com.

NOTE: If you are taking insulin or diabetes medications, or are being treated for a related condition, consult your doctor before taking any supplements.

Blood Type B: Pre-Diabetes/ Metabolic Enhancement Protocol

For support of overall metabolic health and blood sugar regulation		
SUPPLEMENT	**ACTION**	**DOSAGE**
High-potency multivitamin, preferably blood type–specific	Nutritional support	As directed
High-potency mineral complex, preferably blood type–specific	Nutritional support	As directed
Larch arabinogalactan	Promotes intestinal health, excellent fiber source	1 tablespoon, twice daily, in juice or water
Probiotic	Promotes intestinal health	1–2 capsules, twice daily
L-carnitine	Promotes metabolic health, energy, active tissue mass	20 mg daily

SUPPLEMENT	ACTION	DOSAGE
Holy basil (*Ocimum sanctum*)	Improves stress response	500 mg, 1–2 capsules, twice daily
Bromelain	Protein digestive enzyme	500 mg, 1–2 capsules, twice daily

Blood Type B: Type 1 Diabetes Adjunct

Add these supplements for type 1 diabetes		
SUPPLEMENT	ACTION	DOSAGE
Quercetin	Prevents diabetic complications	300–600 mg, twice daily
Zinc	Prevents deficiency common to type 1 diabetics	25 mg daily
Magnesium	Prevents deficiency common to Blood Type B diabetics	200–300 mg daily

Blood Type B: Type 2 Diabetes Adjunct

Add these supplements for type 2 diabetes		
SUPPLEMENT	ACTION	DOSAGE
Quercetin	Prevents diabetic complications	300–600 mg, twice daily
Magnesium	Prevents deficiency common to Blood Type B diabetics	200–300 mg, daily
Fenugreek	Lowers blood sugar, improves glucose tolerance	300–600 mg, twice daily
Asian ginseng	Stabilizes blood sugar and prevents post-meal hyperglycemia	100–300 mg, 40 minutes before eating (avoid if you have high blood pressure)

Blood Type B:
Diabetic Complications Adjunct

SUPPLEMENT	ACTION	DOSAGE
Gotu Kola (*Centella asiatica*)	Improves circulation, promotes wound healing, lowers blood pressure	100 mg, 1–2 capsules, twice daily (do not take if you are pregnant)
Alpha-lipoic acid	Improves diabetic neuropathy and relieves pain	50–100 mg daily
Dandelion (*Taraxacum officinale*)	Reduces edema	250 mg capsule daily, or fresh in salad or tea
Stinging nettle root (*Urtica dioica*)	Reduces edema	500 mg, 1–2 times daily, away from meals

The Exercise Component

FOR BLOOD TYPE B, stress regulation and overall fitness are achieved with a balance of moderate aerobic activity and mentally soothing, stress-reducing exercises. Below is the recommended activity program for Blood Type B.

EXERCISE	DURATION	FREQUENCY
Tennis	45–60 minutes	2–3 x week
Martial arts	30–60 minutes	2–3 x week
Cycling	45–60 minutes	2–3 x week
Hiking	30–60 minutes	2–3 x week
Golf (no cart!)	60–90 minutes	2–3 x week
Running or brisk walking	40–50 minutes	2–3 x week
Pilates	40–50 minutes	2–3 x week
Swimming	45 minutes	2–3 x week

EXERCISE	DURATION	FREQUENCY
Yoga	40–50 minutes	1–2 x week
T'ai Chi	40–50 minutes	1–2 x week

3 Steps to Effective Exercise

1. Before you begin your aerobic exercise, warm up with a walk. Then perform some careful stretching movements to increase flexibility.
2. To achieve maximum cardiovascular benefits, work toward an elevated heart rate that is about 70 percent of your capacity. Once you reach the elevated rate, continue exercising to maintain that rate for twenty to thirty minutes. To calculate your maximum heart rate and performance level:
   - Subtract your age from 220.
   - Multiply the difference by .70 (or .60 if you are over age sixty). This is the high end of your performance.
   - Multiply the remainder by .50. This is the low end of your performance.
3. Finish each aerobic session with at least a five-minute cooldown, combining some careful stretching and flexibility movements with a relaxing walk.

Getting Started: The First Month

IF YOU ARE NEW to the Blood Type Diet and exercise plan, the following guidelines will introduce you to the Blood Type B regimen over a period of one month. Follow these recommendations as closely as possible, using a journal to record your personal experience with the diet. In addition to measurable factors, such as weight loss, blood sugar regulation, and blood pressure, take the time to note changes in energy levels, sleep patterns, mood, and overall well-being. Over time you'll learn to manage your diet and exercise patterns to achieve the maximum results.

Blood Type B Diabetes Diet Checklist

Eat small to moderate portions of high-quality, lean, organic ☐
meat several times a week for strength, energy, and efficient
metabolism.

If you are not used to eating dairy products, introduce them ☐
gradually, after you have been on the Blood Type B Diet for several weeks. Begin with cultured dairy products, such as yogurt
and kefir, which are more easily tolerated than fresh dairy
products.

Include regular portions of richly oiled cold-water fish. Fish oils ☐
can boost your metabolism.

Eliminate wheat and wheat-based products from your diet, if ☐
you have weight or blood sugar problems.

Avoid foods that promote insulin resistance. For Blood Type B ☐
these include buckwheat, chicken, corn, lentils, peanuts,
sesame seeds, and tomatoes.

Eat lots of BENEFICIAL fruits and vegetables. ☐

Don't undereat or skip meals. Use appropriate blood type ☐
snacks between meals if you get hungry. Avoid low-calorie
diets. Remember, food deprivation is a huge stress. It raises
cortisol levels, lowers metabolism, encourages fat storage, and
depletes healthy muscle mass.

Limit sugar, caffeine, and alcohol. These are short-term "fixes" ☐
that ultimately increase stress and slow down your metabolism.

Week 1

Blood Type Diet and Supplements

- Cut back or eliminate your most harmful AVOID foods—chicken, corn, and
  buckwheat. These foods seriously interfere with proper metabolism.

- Include your most important BENEFICIAL foods at least five times this week. These include lamb, seafood, and cultured dairy.

- Incorporate at least one SUPER BENEFICIAL food into your daily diet. For example, have a handful of walnuts as a snack, or eat yogurt mixed with berries for lunch.

- If you're a heavy coffee drinker, begin to wean yourself by cutting your daily consumption in half. Substitute a high-quality green tea, such as Itaru's Premium Green Tea, which is available from our Web site.

- To improve blood sugar regulation, eat 5 to 6 small meals throughout the day, rather than 3 large meals.

- If you are taking insulin or diabetes medications, speak with your doctor before taking supplements; your dosages may need to be changed.

Exercise Regimen

- Plan to exercise at least 4 days this week, for 45 minutes each day.
  2–3 days: aerobic activity
  1–2 days: yoga or T'ai Chi

- Use your journal to detail the time, activity, distance, and amount of weight. Note the repetitions used for each exercise.

▪ WEEK 1 SUCCESS STRATEGY ▪

High stress levels will undermine your efforts to regulate blood sugar. Take advantage of Blood Type B's natural ability to relieve stress through meditation or guided imagery. Of all the meditation techniques, "TM," or transcendental meditation, has been the most thoroughly studied for its antistress effects. Evidence indicates that cortisol decreases during meditation—especially for long-term practitioners—and remains somewhat lower after meditation. Set aside 20 to 30 minutes every day to meditate.

Week 2

Blood Type Diet and Supplements

- Begin to eliminate the next level of AVOID foods—seeds, beans, and legumes.

- Eat at least one BENEFICIAL animal protein every day.

- Initially, it is best to avoid foods on the NEUTRAL: Allowed Infrequently list. After a few weeks, if your condition improves, you may have them once or twice a month.

- Continue to incorporate SUPER BENEFICIAL foods into your daily diet.
- If you're a coffee drinker, continue to cut your coffee intake, replacing it with Itaru's Premium Green Tea.
- Continue to eat 5 to 6 small meals throughout the day, rather than 3 large meals.

▪ WEEK 2 SUCCESS STRATEGY ▪

Don't leave home without a quick snack tucked into your purse or briefcase to offset low blood sugar.
   Suggestions:

- Super Smoothie in a Thermos, made with 2 tablespoons whey-based protein powder, 1 banana, 1 papaya, and ½ cup pineapple juice
- Trail mix: dried banana, dried cherries, walnuts, almonds
- Cup of yogurt with berries

Exercise Regimen

- Continue to exercise at least 4 days this week, for 45 minutes each day.
   2–3 days: aerobic activity
   1–2 days: yoga or T'ai Chi

Week 3

Blood Type Diet and Supplements

- When you plan your meals for week 3, choose BENEFICIAL foods to replace NEUTRAL foods whenever possible. For example, choose lamb over beef, or a plum over an apple.
- Eliminate all remaining AVOID foods.
- Liberally incorporate SUPER BENEFICIAL foods into your daily diet.
- Completely wean yourself from coffee, substituting Itaru's Premium Green Tea.
- Continue to eat 5 to 6 small meals throughout the day, rather than 3 large meals.
- Drink a cup of licorice tea (DGL licorice) after meals to lower blood sugar.

Exercise Regimen

- Continue to exercise at least 4 days this week, for 45 minutes each day.
   2–3 days: aerobic activity

1–2 days: yoga or T'ai Chi

- Add one day of unstructured exercise—walking, biking, swimming.

■ WEEK 3 SUCCESS STRATEGY ■

Fight carbohydrate cravings. If you crave any form of stimulants or carbohydrates, your serotonin levels are low, and your brain is demanding stimulants to raise your serotonin levels.

Try a sip of vegetable glycerine between meals to cut down on your cravings. For women, low estrogen levels can produce carbohydrate craving. One or two capsules of the herb maca can help normalize your estrogen levels.

Week 4

Blood Type Diet and Supplements

- Continue at the week 3 level, focusing on BENEFICIAL and SUPER BENEFICIAL foods.

- Continue to eat 5 to 6 small meals throughout the day, rather than 3 large meals.

- Evaluate your progress during the first three weeks and make adjustments.

Exercise Regimen

- Continue at the week 3 level.

- Evaluate your progress, referring to your journal. Determine which exercise regimen has worked for you, including time of day, setting, and activity level. Look for ways to improve your performance and endurance.

■ WEEK 4 SUCCESS STRATEGY ■

Maintaining a regular sleep cycle is crucial to the reduction of stress and the maintenance of an efficient metabolism. Reestablishing your circadian rhythm—important for control of cortisol levels—can be difficult for seniors. Overall, elderly people tend to have more problems with interrupted sleep and insomnia. You may need to increase your intake of vitamin B_{12} or take a melatonin supplement.

FAQs: Blood Type B and Diabetes

My blood pressure tends to be slightly high. I am working to control it with diet, so I don't have to take medications. Are there any natural remedies for Type B?

Insulin-resistant Blood Type Bs are somewhat more susceptible to high blood pressure. The good news is that Blood Type B individuals seem to have a remarkable capacity for reducing stress by practicing visualization and relaxation techniques. In my practice, I never attempt to treat a Type B who has high blood pressure with medications until I first suggest that the patient try using relaxation and visualization. More often than not, simple visualization techniques work as well as, or better than, hypertension meds.

Here's a food-based suggestion: Juice several stalks of celery (enough to produce 6–8 ounces of juice) and drink it daily. It's an excellent tonic for blood pressure regulation.

Finally, an excellent technique for alleviating stress and balancing the nervous system is alternate nostril breathing. Left nostril breathing generates a more relaxing effect. Right nostril breathing generates a more energized effect. Switching back and forth tends to balance your nervous system. Holding your right nostril closed, breathe slowly through the left nostril to the count of ten. Switch nostrils and repeat. Perform the exercise five times.

I am Blood Type B. I have always had problems digesting dairy foods, and I may be lactose intolerant. What can I do?

Slowly introduce dairy foods. Use a "lactase," or lactose-digestive, enzyme preparation for the first few weeks of eating dairy. It should make dairy foods easier to digest, and you can then slowly wean yourself off the lactase. Start with cultured dairy foods, such as yogurt, before you move to fresh milk products. Simultaneously, make the other adjustments in your diet—emphasizing as many BENEFICIAL foods as possible, and avoiding the foods that are difficult for you to digest. I've found that lactose-intolerant Type Bs find dairy surprisingly friendly once they have made the other changes to their diets.

**My three-year-old has type 1 diabetes, and she's a very fussy eater.
I worry that she won't get the nutrients she needs.**

Young children with diabetes can go through the same fussy eating phases as other children. It's usually best not to force a fussy child to eat. Have a variety of foods available. If the child rejects one food, offer something else, or offer juice or milk instead. The American Diabetes Association offers many tips for parenting children with diabetes on its Web site.

**I see that watermelon is SUPER BENEFICIAL for Blood Type B,
but it is also high on the glycemic index. Shouldn't I avoid it?**

This is a clear example of the reason why food recommendations must be individualized. Although watermelon is high on the glycemic index, it moderates insulin's effects and reduces edema for Blood Type B, especially non-secretors.

**I am new to the Blood Type Diet, and since I have not been a meat
eater for several years, I'm having a hard time adjusting to the
meat in the Type B diet.**

You need to make your dietary changes gradually. The protein in your diet should emphasize a combination of seafood and dairy, with very limited amounts of BENEFICIAL meats, such as lamb. Until you have adapted to the diet, stay away from some of the NEUTRAL meats, such as beef, veal, liver, and pheasant. Take a "pancreatic enzyme" (available in most health-food stores) with your main meal until you adapt to eating meat and dairy. Bromelain, an enzyme found in pineapple, is another helpful supplement. In addition, ginger, peppermint, and parsley are all good stomach tonics.

A Final Word

IN SUMMARY, the secret to fighting diabetes with the Blood Type B Diet involves:

1. Increasing active tissue mass (calorie-burning tissue) by switching to a more animal protein–based diet.
2. Minimizing consumption of the insulin-mimicking lectins, abundant in grains such as wheat and corn.
3. Increasing circulatory efficiency, lowering triglycerides and blood pressure, and reducing cortisol by adopting an exercise strategy that combines calming activities with vigorous routines.
4. Using supplements intelligently to block the effect of insulin-mimicking lectins, provide antioxidant support, and protect delicate nerve tissue from destruction.

SEVEN

Blood Type

AB

BLOOD TYPE AB HAS A MIXED PROFILE WHEN IT COMES TO diabetes risk factors. Like Blood Type A, you are more likely to have cardiovascular complications due to diabetes, as well as complications related to blood clotting. However, like Blood Type B, you are highly sensitive to certain insulin-mimicking lectins.

Although you need a bit more animal protein in your diet than Blood Type A, you lack enough stomach acid to digest large amounts of it efficiently. Similarly, you have some difficulty metabolizing combinations of protein and fat, due to your low levels of intestinal alkaline phosphatase.

Because you also share some B-specific characteristics, you must also be careful to avoid insulin-mimicking lectins that react with the B antigen. Overall, the best guideline for Blood Type AB is to draw from the best of both A and B worlds.

Blood Type Weight Profile

Weight Gain		Weight Loss	
FOOD	**MECHANISM**	**FOOD**	**MECHANISM**
Chicken	Promotes insulin resistance	Soy	Optimizes metabolism and aids digestion
Red meat	Poorly digested and stored as fat	Seafood	Helps regulate blood sugar
Kidney beans, lima beans	Promote insulin resistance	Cultured dairy	Improves insulin response
Buckwheat	Promotes insulin resistance and impairs calorie utilization	Broccoli, greens	Improve metabolic efficiency
Processed sugar	Promotes insulin resistance	Cherries, plums	Improve insulin response

Special Risks for Non-Secretors

IF YOU ARE A BLOOD TYPE AB non-secretor, you have an even greater risk of developing diabetes and of developing complications from diabetes.

From a statistical standpoint alone, non-secretors are three times more likely than secretors to become diabetic. Overall, Blood Type AB non-secretors have a higher risk of all conditions associated with Metabolic Syndrome, including high cholesterol, hypertension, and insulin resistance.

Research shows that several of the risk factors associated with the A antigen become magnified when you are a non-secretor. The activity of intestinal alkaline phosphatase, which is involved in fat digestion, is already low in Blood Type AB, and is even lower in non-secretors. If you are a Type A non-secretor, your alkaline phosphatase activity is only about 20 percent that of secretors. Being a non-secretor also has an impact on blood-clotting ability. Blood Type AB tends to have raised levels of certain clotting factors, contributing to their risk for heart disease and thrombosis. If you are also a non-secretor, your clotting factors are generally even higher.

Taken together, these factors can make a big difference for a Blood Type AB individual, so it's important that you find out your secretor status. (See Appendix B for information about ordering a saliva test.)

Blood Type AB: The Foods

THE BLOOD TYPE AB Diabetes Diet is specifically adapted for the prevention and management of diabetes. The new category, **Super Beneficial**, highlights powerful diabetes-fighting foods for Blood Type AB. The **Neutral** category has also been adjusted to de-emphasize foods that can cause problems for diabetics. Foods designated **Neutral: Allowed Infrequently** should be minimized or avoided entirely, depending on your condition. Eat these foods no more than once or twice a month. Your secretor status can influence your ability to fully digest and metabolize certain foods, so some adjustments in the values are made for non-secretors. If you do not know your secretor type, the odds are that you can safely use the "secretor" values, since the majority of the population (80 percent) are secretors. However, I urge you to get tested, since the variations are important for non-secretors who want to maximize the effectiveness of the Blood Type Diet.

The food charts are divided into three sections. The top of the chart suggests the average portion size and quantity per week or day, according to secretor status. These recommendations do *not* apply to the category **Neutral: Allowed Infrequently**; those foods should be consumed sparingly (0–2 times a month). The charts also indicate differences in frequency based on ethnic heritage. It has been my experience that this factor has an impact on the individual's ability to fully digest certain foods. For the purposes of blood type food choices, persons of Hispanic heritage should follow the recommendations for Caucasians, and North American Native peoples should follow the recommendations for Asians.

The middle section of the chart provides the food values. The bottom section lists variants based on secretor status.

For your convenience, we have included a number of product names, such as ketchup, Worcestershire sauce, and Ezekiel bread. However, bear in mind that commercial formulations vary among brands and regions. Even though a product may be listed as okay for you, always check its ingredients; do not use products that contain **Avoid** ingredients for your blood type. Of course, you may choose to make your own version of commercial products such as bread and mayonnaise, using ingredients that suit your blood type. There are hundreds of delicious recipes for every blood type available on our Web site (www.dadamo.com) or in the book *Cook Right 4 Your Type: The Practical Kitchen Companion to* Eat Right 4 Your Type.

Food Values

SUPER BENEFICIAL	Foods that are known to have specific disease-fighting qualities for your blood type.
BENEFICIAL	Foods with components that enhance the metabolic, immune, or structural health of your blood type.
NEUTRAL: Allowed Frequently	Foods that normally have no direct blood type effect but supply a variety of nutrients necessary for a healthful diet.
NEUTRAL: Allowed Infrequently	Foods that normally have no blood type effect but may impede your progress when consumed regularly.
AVOID	Foods with components that are harmful to your blood type.

Meat/Poultry

Although a bit better adapted to animal-based proteins than Blood Type A (mainly because of your B gene's effects on digestive secretions), Blood Type AB still has to be aware of the tendency for elevated cholesterol—a problem of somewhat less concern if you are a non-secretor. Emphasize free-range, chemical-, antobiotic-, and pesticide-free, low-fat meats and poultry.

BLOOD TYPE AB: MEAT/POULTRY			
Portion: 4–6 oz (men); 2–5 oz (women and children)			
	African	Caucasian	Asian
Secretor	2–5	1–5	1–5
Non-Secretor	3–5	2–5	2–5
		Times per week	

SUPER BENEFICIAL	BENEFICIAL	NEUTRAL: Allowed Frequently	NEUTRAL: Allowed Infrequently	AVOID
	Lamb	Goat	Liver (calf)	All commercially processed meats
	Mutton	Ostrich		Bacon/Ham/Pork
	Rabbit	Pheasant		Beef
	Turkey			Buffalo
				Chicken
				Cornish hen
				Duck
				Goose
				Grouse
				Guinea hen
				Heart (beef)
				Horse
				Partridge
				Quail
				Squab
				Squirrel
				Sweetbreads
				Turtle

SUPER BENEFICIAL	BENEFICIAL	NEUTRAL: Allowed Frequently	NEUTRAL: Allowed Infrequently	AVOID
				Veal
				Venison
Special Variants: *Non-Secretor* NEUTRAL (Allowed Frequently): quail, venison.				

Fish/Seafood

Fish and seafood represent an excellent source of protein for Blood Type AB individuals, increasing active tissue mass and providing arterial, sugar metabolism, cardiac, and nervous system support through their stimulation of docosahexaenoic acid (DHA) production.

BLOOD TYPE AB: FISH/SEAFOOD			
Portion: 4–6 oz (men); 2–5 oz (women and children)			
	African	Caucasian	Asian
Secretor	4–6	3–5	3–5
Non-Secretor	4–7	4–6	4–6
		Times per week	

SUPER BENEFICIAL	BENEFICIAL	NEUTRAL: Allowed Frequently	NEUTRAL: Allowed Infrequently	AVOID
Cod	Grouper	Abalone	Caviar	Anchovy
Mackerel	Mahi-mahi	Bluefish	(sturgeon)	Barracuda
Red	Monkfish	Bullhead	Mussels	Bass (all)
snapper	Pickerel	Butterfish	Scallop	Beluga
Salmon	Pike	Carp	Squid (calamari)	Clam
Sardine	Porgy	Catfish	Whitefish	Conch
	Sailfish	Chub		Crab
	Shad	Croaker		Eel
	Snail	Cusk		Flounder
	(*Helix pomatia*/ escargot)	Drum		Frog
		Halfmoon fish		Gray sole
				Haddock

SUPER BENEFICIAL	BENEFICIAL	NEUTRAL: Allowed Frequently	NEUTRAL: Allowed Infrequently	AVOID
	Sturgeon	Harvest fish		Hake
	Tuna	Herring (fresh)		Halibut
		Mullet		Herring (pickled/ smoked)
		Muskellunge		Lobster
		Opaleye		Octopus
		Orange roughy		Oysters
		Parrot fish		Salmon (smoked)
		Perch (all)		Salmon roe
		Pollock		Shrimp
		Pompano		Sole
		Rosefish		Trout (all)
		Scrod		Whiting
		Scup		Yellowtail
		Shark		
		Smelt		
		Sucker		
		Sunfish		
		Swordfish		
		Tilapia		
		Tilefish		
		Tuna		
		Weakfish		

Special Variants: *Non-Secretor* BENEFICIAL: herring (fresh); NEUTRAL (Allowed Frequently): trout (all).

Dairy/Eggs

Dairy products confer benefits on Blood Type AB individuals, especially secretors. Eggs, another good source of DHA, can complement the protein profile for your blood type and help you build active tissue mass. If you are of African ancestry, you may need to minimize non-cultured forms of dairy, such as whole milk and cheese. Do your best to find eggs and dairy products that meet organic standards.

BLOOD TYPE AB: EGGS

Portion: 1 egg

	African	Caucasian	Asian
Secretor	2–5	3–4	3–4
Non-Secretor	3–6	3–6	3–6
		Times per week	

BLOOD TYPE AB: MILK AND YOGURT

Portion: 4–6 oz (men); 2–5 oz (women and children)

	African	Caucasian	Asian
Secretor	2–6	3–6	1–6
Non-Secretor	0–3	0–4	0–3
		Times per week	

BLOOD TYPE AB: CHEESE

Portion: 3 oz (men); 2 oz (women and children)

	African	Caucasian	Asian
Secretor	2–3	3–4	3–4
Non-Secretor	0	0–1	0
		Times per week	

SUPER BENEFICIAL	BENEFICIAL	NEUTRAL: Allowed Frequently	NEUTRAL: Allowed Infrequently	AVOID
Kefir	Cottage cheese	Casein	Cheddar	American cheese
Milk (goat)	Egg (chicken)	Cream cheese	Colby	Blue cheese
Yogurt	Farmer cheese	Edam	Emmenthal	Brie
	Feta	Egg (goose/quail)	Ghee (clarified butter)	Butter
	Goat cheese	Gouda	Milk (cow)	Buttermilk
	Mozzarella	Gruyère	Monterey Jack	Camembert
	Ricotta	Jarlsberg	Sherbet	Egg (duck)
	Sour cream	Muenster	Swiss cheese	Half-and-half
		Neufchâtel		Ice cream
		Paneer		Parmesan
				Provolone

SUPER BENEFICIAL	BENEFICIAL	NEUTRAL: Allowed Frequently	NEUTRAL: Allowed Infrequently	AVOID
		Quark cheese		
		String cheese		
		Whey		

Special Variants: *Non-Secretor* BENEFICIAL: ghee (clarified butter); NEUTRAL (Allowed Frequently): goat cheese, yogurt; AVOID: Emmenthal, Swiss cheese.

Oils

In general, Blood Type AB does best on monounsaturated oils (such as olive oil) and oils rich in omega series fatty acids (such as flax oil). Non-secretors have a bit of an edge over secretors in breaking down oils, and probably benefit more from their consumption, as these oils enhance the absorption of calcium via the small intestine.

BLOOD TYPE AB: OILS			
Portion: 1 tblsp			
	African	Caucasian	Asian
Secretor	4–7	5–8	5–7
Non-Secretor	3–6	3–6	3–4
		Times per week	

SUPER BENEFICIAL	BENEFICIAL	NEUTRAL: Allowed Frequently	NEUTRAL: Allowed Infrequently	AVOID
	Olive	Almond	Wheat germ	Coconut
	Walnut	Black cur-rant seed		Corn
		Borage seed		Cottonseed
		Canola		Safflower
		Castor		Sesame
		Cod liver		Sunflower

SUPER BENEFICIAL	BENEFICIAL	NEUTRAL: Allowed Frequently	NEUTRAL: Allowed Infrequently	AVOID
		Evening primrose		
		Flax (linseed)		
		Peanut		
		Soy		

Nuts and Seeds

Nuts and seeds are a good secondary protein source for Blood Type AB. Several nuts, such as walnuts, can help lower toxic concentrations in the intestine and are also known to improve blood sugar regulation.

BLOOD TYPE AB: NUTS AND SEEDS			
Portion: Whole (handful); Nut Butters (2 tblsp)			
	African	Caucasian	Asian
Secretor	4–8	4–9	5–9
Non-Secretor	5–10	5–10	5–9
			Times per week

SUPER BENEFICIAL	BENEFICIAL	NEUTRAL: Allowed Frequently	NEUTRAL: Allowed Infrequently	AVOID
Peanut	Chestnut	Almond	Brazil nut	Filbert (hazelnut)
Peanut butter		Almond butter	Cashew	Poppy seed
Walnut (black/ English)		Almond cheese	Cashew butter	Pumpkin seed
		Almond milk	Macadamia	Sesame butter (tahini)
		Beechnut	Pecan	
		Butternut	Pecan butter	Sesame seed
			Pistachio	

SUPER BENEFICIAL	BENEFICIAL	NEUTRAL: Allowed Frequently	NEUTRAL: Allowed Infrequently	AVOID
		Flax (linseed) Hickory Litchi Pignolia (pine nut)	Safflower seed	Sunflower butter Sunflower seed

Special Variants: *Non-Secretor* NEUTRAL (Allowed Frequently): peanut, peanut butter; AVOID: Brazil, cashew, pistachio.

Beans and Legumes

Blood Type AB does well on proteins found in many beans and legumes, although this food category contains more than a few beans with problematic A- or B-specific lectins. In general, this category is only marginally sufficient to build active tissue mass in Blood Type AB, and even less so for non-secretors.

BLOOD TYPE AB: BEANS AND LEGUMES			
Portion: 1 cup (cooked)			
	African	Caucasian	Asian
Secretor	3–6	3–6	4–6
Non-Secretor	2–5	2–5	3–6
		Times per week	

SUPER BENEFICIAL	BENEFICIAL	NEUTRAL: Allowed Frequently	NEUTRAL: Allowed Infrequently	AVOID
Miso Soy bean Tempeh Tofu	Lentil (green) Navy bean Pinto bean	Bean (green/ snap/ string) Cannellini bean	Jicama bean	Adzuki bean Black bean Black-eyed pea Fava (broad) bean

SUPER BENEFICIAL	BENEFICIAL	NEUTRAL: Allowed Frequently	NEUTRAL: Allowed Infrequently	AVOID
		Copper bean		Garbanzo (chickpea)
		Lentil (domestic/red)		Kidney bean
		Northern bean		Lima bean
		Pea (green/pod/snow)		Mung bean/sprout
		Soy cheese		
		Soy milk		
		Tamarind bean		
		White bean		

Special Variants: *Non-Secretor* NEUTRAL (Allowed Frequently): fava (broad) bean, miso, navy bean, soy bean, tempeh, tofu; AVOID: jicama bean, soy cheese, soy milk.

Grains and Starches

Blood Type AB secretors have many choices of grains. Bear in mind that wheat is not a very good choice for Blood Type AB, especially non-secretors. The wheat lectin can exert an insulin-like effect on your body, lowering active tissue mass and increasing total body fat.

BLOOD TYPE AB: GRAINS AND STARCHES			
Portion: ½ cup dry (grains or pastas); 1 muffin; 2 slices of bread			
	African	Caucasian	Asian
Secretor	6–8	6–9	6–10
Non-Secretor	4–6	5–7	6–8
		Times per week	

SUPER BENEFICIAL	BENEFICIAL	NEUTRAL: Allowed Frequently	NEUTRAL: Allowed Infrequently	AVOID
	Amaranth	Barley	Wheat (bran)	Buckwheat
	Essene bread (Manna)	Couscous	Wheat (semolina)	Cornmeal
	Ezekiel 4:9 bread	Spelt flour/products	Wheat (whole)	Grits
	Millet	Quinoa	Wheat germ	Kamut
	Oat bran			Popcorn
	Oat flour			Soba noodles (100% buckwheat)
	Oatmeal			Sorghum
	Rice (whole)			Tapioca
	Rice (wild)			Teff
	Rice bran			Wheat (refined unbleached)
	Rice cake			Wheat (white flour)
	Rye (whole)			
	Rye flour/products			
	Soy flour/products			
	Spelt (whole)			

Special Variants: *Non-Secretor* NEUTRAL (Allowed Frequently): Ezekiel 4:9 bread, spelt (whole); AVOID: soy flour/products, wheat (germ), wheat (semolina), wheat (whole).

Vegetables

Vegetables provide a rich source of antioxidants and fiber, and also help to lower the production of toxins in the digestive tract. Many vegetables are rich in potassium, helping to reduce water retention. Mushrooms are great for Blood Type AB diabetics. Research shows that the mushroom lectin (*Agaricus bisporus*) stimulates insulin release from the pancreas and aids in proper insulin regulation. An item's value also applies to its juice, unless otherwise noted.

BLOOD TYPE AB: VEGETABLES

Portion: 1 cup prepared (cooked or raw)

	African	Caucasian	Asian
Secretor	Unlimited	Unlimited	Unlimited
Non-Secretor	Unlimited	Unlimited	Unlimited
		Times per day	

SUPER BENEFICIAL	BENEFICIAL	NEUTRAL: Allowed Frequently	NEUTRAL: Allowed Infrequently	AVOID
Beet	Alfalfa	Arugula	Carrot	Aloe
Beet greens	sprout	Asparagus	Daikon	Artichoke
Broccoli	Cabbage	Asparagus	radish	Corn
Collard	(juice)*	pea	Olive	Mushroom
Kale	Carrot	Bamboo	(Greek/	(abalone/
Mushroom	(juice)	shoot	green/	shiitake)
(maitake)	Cauli-	Bean	Spanish)	Olive (black)
Mustard	flower	(green/	Poi	Pepper (all)
greens	Celery	snap/	Potato	Pickle (all)
	Cucumber	string)	Pumpkin	Radish/
	Dandelion	Bok choy	Taro	sprouts
	Eggplant	Brussels		Rhubarb
	Garlic	sprout		
	Parsnip	Cabbage		
	Potato	Celeriac		
	(sweet)	Chicory		
	Yam	Cucumber		
		(juice)*		
		Endive		
		Escarole		
		Fennel		
		Fiddlehead		
		fern		
		Horseradish		
		Kohlrabi		
		Leek		
		Lettuce (all)		

SUPER BENEFICIAL	BENEFICIAL	NEUTRAL: Allowed Frequently	NEUTRAL: Allowed Infrequently	AVOID
		Mushroom (enoki/ oyster/ portobello/ silver dollar/ straw/ tree ear)		
		Okra		
		Onion (all)		
		Oyster plant		
		Pea (green/ pod/snow)		
		Radicchio		
		Rappini (broccoli rabe)		
		Rutabaga		
		Scallion		
		Seaweed		
		Shallot		
		Spinach		
		Squash (all)		
		Swiss chard		
		Tomato		
		Turnip		
		Water chestnut		
		Watercress		
		Yucca		
		Zucchini		

Special Variants: *Non-Secretor* BENEFICIAL: tomato; NEUTRAL (Allowed Frequently): beet; AVOID: poi, taro.

*To obtain the benefits of cabbage and cucumber juice, they must be consumed within one minute of juicing.

Fruits and Fruit Juices

Fruits are rich in antioxidants, and many, such as blueberries, elderberries, cherries, and blackberries, contain polysaccharides that block the liver enzyme ornithine decarboxylase (ODC). This has the effect of lowering the production of chemicals that act with insulin to encourage weight gain.

A diet rich in proper fruits and vegetables can help weight loss by tempering the effects of insulin while also helping to shift the balance of water in the body from high extracellular concentrations (edema) to high intracellular concentrations. Many fruits, such as pineapple, are rich in enzymes that can help reduce inflammation and encourage proper water balance. Non-secretors have somewhat reduced portion frequencies and a number of food value changes in this category.

An item's value also applies to its juice, unless otherwise noted.

BLOOD TYPE AB: FRUITS AND FRUIT JUICES			
Portion: 1 cup			
	African	Caucasian	Asian
Secretor	3–4	3–6	3–5
Non-Secretor	1–3	2–3	3–4
		Times per day	

SUPER BENEFICIAL	BENEFICIAL	NEUTRAL: Allowed Frequently	NEUTRAL: Allowed Infrequently	AVOID
Cherry	Fig (fresh/ dried)	Apple	Apricot	Avocado
Cranberry	Gooseberry	Blackberry	Asian pear	Banana
Pineapple	Grape (all)	Blueberry	Breadfruit	Bitter melon
Water- melon	Grapefruit	Boysen- berry	Canang melon	Coconut
	Kiwi	Elderberry (dark blue/ purple)	Cantaloupe	Dewberry
	Lemon		Casaba melon	Guava
	Logan- berry	Grapefruit (juice)	Christmas melon	Loganberry
	Plum			Mango
				Orange
				Persimmon

SUPER BENEFICIAL	BENEFICIAL	NEUTRAL: Allowed Frequently	NEUTRAL: Allowed Infrequently	AVOID
		Kumquat	Crenshaw melon	Pomegranate
		Lime	Currant	Prickly pear
		Mulberry	Date	Quince
		Muskmelon	Honeydew	Sago palm
		Nectarine	Prune	Star fruit (carambola)
		Papaya	Raisin	
		Peach	Tangerine	
		Pear		
		Persian melon		
		Pineapple (juice)		
		Plantain		
		Raspberry		
		Spanish melon		
		Strawberry		
		Youngberry		

Special Variants: *Non-Secretor* BENEFICIAL: blackberry, blueberry, elderberry, lime; NEUTRAL (Allowed Frequently): banana; AVOID: cantaloupe, honeydew, prune, tangerine.

Spices/Condiments/Sweeteners

Many spices have mild to moderate medicinal properties, often because of their influence on bacterial populations in the lower intestine. Turmeric contains a powerful phytochemical called curcumin, which lowers levels of intestinal toxins. Brewer's yeast is a beneficial food for Blood Type AB non-secretors, enhancing glucose metabolism and helping to ensure a healthy flora balance in the intestinal tract. Many common food additives, such as guar gum and carrageenan, should be avoided as they can enhance the effects of lectins found in other foods.

SUPER BENEFICIAL	BENEFICIAL	NEUTRAL: Allowed Frequently	NEUTRAL: Allowed Infrequently	AVOID
Ginger Turmeric	Garlic Horseradish Molasses (blackstrap) Oregano Parsley	Basil Bay leaf Bergamot Caraway Cardamom Carob Chervil Chili powder Chive Cilantro (coriander leaf) Cinnamon Clove Coriander Cream of tartar Cumin Dill Juniper Licorice root* Mace Marjoram Mint (all) Mustard (dry) Nutmeg Paprika Rosemary Saffron Sage Savory Sea salt Seaweed	Agar Apple pectin Arrowroot Chocolate Honey Maple syrup Mayonnaise Molasses Rice syrup Soy sauce Sugar (brown/ white)	Allspice Almond extract Anise Aspartame Barley malt Carrageenan Cornstarch Corn syrup Dextrose Fructose Gelatin (except veg-sourced) Guarana Gums (acacia/Arabic guar) Ketchup Maltodextrin MSG Pepper (black/ white/ peppercorn/red flakes) Pepper (cayenne) Pickle (all) Sucanat Tapioca Vinegar (all) Worcestershire sauce

SUPER BENEFICIAL	BENEFICIAL	NEUTRAL: Allowed Frequently	NEUTRAL: Allowed Infrequently	AVOID
		Kumquat	Crenshaw melon	Pomegranate
		Lime	Currant	Prickly pear
		Mulberry	Date	Quince
		Muskmelon	Honeydew	Sago palm
		Nectarine	Prune	Star fruit (carambola)
		Papaya	Raisin	
		Peach	Tangerine	
		Pear		
		Persian melon		
		Pineapple (juice)		
		Plantain		
		Raspberry		
		Spanish melon		
		Strawberry		
		Youngberry		

Special Variants: *Non-Secretor* BENEFICIAL: blackberry, blueberry, elderberry, lime; NEUTRAL (Allowed Frequently): banana; AVOID: cantaloupe, honeydew, prune, tangerine.

Spices/Condiments/Sweeteners

Many spices have mild to moderate medicinal properties, often because of their influence on bacterial populations in the lower intestine. Turmeric contains a powerful phytochemical called curcumin, which lowers levels of intestinal toxins. Brewer's yeast is a beneficial food for Blood Type AB non-secretors, enhancing glucose metabolism and helping to ensure a healthy flora balance in the intestinal tract. Many common food additives, such as guar gum and carrageenan, should be avoided as they can enhance the effects of lectins found in other foods.

SUPER BENEFICIAL	BENEFICIAL	NEUTRAL: Allowed Frequently	NEUTRAL: Allowed Infrequently	AVOID
Ginger	Garlic	Basil	Agar	Allspice
Turmeric	Horserad-	Bay leaf	Apple	Almond
	ish	Bergamot	pectin	extract
	Molasses	Caraway	Arrowroot	Anise
	(black-	Cardamom	Chocolate	Aspartame
	strap)	Carob	Honey	Barley malt
	Oregano	Chervil	Maple	Carrageenan
	Parsley	Chili	syrup	Cornstarch
		powder	Mayon-	Corn syrup
		Chive	naise	Dextrose
		Cilantro	Molasses	Fructose
		(coriander	Rice syrup	Gelatin (ex-
		leaf)	Soy sauce	cept veg-
		Cinnamon	Sugar	sourced)
		Clove	(brown/	Guarana
		Coriander	white)	Gums (aca-
		Cream of		cia/Arabic
		tartar		guar)
		Cumin		Ketchup
		Dill		Maltodex-
		Juniper		trin
		Licorice		MSG
		root*		Pepper
		Mace		(black/
		Marjoram		white/
		Mint (all)		pepper-
		Mustard		corn/red
		(dry)		flakes)
		Nutmeg		Pepper
		Paprika		(cayenne)
		Rosemary		Pickle (all)
		Saffron		Sucanat
		Sage		Tapioca
		Savory		Vinegar
		Sea salt		(all)
		Seaweed		Worcester-
				shire sauce

SUPER BENEFICIAL	BENEFICIAL	NEUTRAL: Allowed Frequently	NEUTRAL: Allowed Infrequently	AVOID
		Senna		
		Stevia		
		Tamari (wheat-free)		
		Tamarind		
		Tarragon		
		Thyme		
		Vanilla		
		Wintergreen		
		Yeast (baker's/brewer's)		

Special Variants: *Non-Secretor* BENEFICIAL: bay leaf, yeast (brewer's); NEUTRAL (Allowed Frequently): miso; AVOID: agar, honey, juniper, maple syrup, rice syrup, sugar (brown/white).

*Avoid if you have high blood pressure.

Herbal Teas

SUPER BENEFICIAL	BENEFICIAL	NEUTRAL: Allowed Frequently	NEUTRAL: Allowed Infrequently	AVOID
Dandelion	Alfalfa	Catnip	Senna	Aloe
Ginseng	Burdock	Chickweed		Coltsfoot
Licorice root*	Chamomile	Dong Quai		Corn silk
	Echinacea	Elder		Fenugreek
	Ginger	Goldenseal		Gentian
	Hawthorn	Horehound		Hops
	Parsley	Mulberry		Linden
	Rosehip	Peppermint		Mullein
	Strawberry leaf	Raspberry leaf		Red clover
		Sage		Rhubarb
		Sarsaparilla		Shepherd's purse

SUPER BENEFICIAL	BENEFICIAL	NEUTRAL: Allowed Frequently	NEUTRAL: Allowed Infrequently	AVOID
		Slippery elm		Skullcap
		Spearmint		
		St. John's wort		
		Thyme		
		Valerian		
		Vervain		
		White birch		
		White oak bark		
		Yarrow		
		Yellow dock		

*Avoid if you have high blood pressure.

Miscellaneous Beverages

You may wish to have a glass of red wine occasionally with your meals; you derive substantial benefit to the cardiovascular system from moderate use. Green tea should be part of every Blood Type AB's health plan.

SUPER BENEFICIAL	BENEFICIAL	NEUTRAL: Allowed Frequently	NEUTRAL: Allowed Infrequently	AVOID
Tea (green)	Wine (red)	Beer		Coffee (reg/decaf)
		Seltzer		Liquor
		Soda (club)		Soda (cola/diet/misc.)
		Wine (white)		Tea, black (reg/decaf)

Special Variants: *Non-Secretor* NEUTRAL (Allowed Frequently): liquor; AVOID: beer.

Supplement Protocols

THE DIET FOR BLOOD TYPE AB offers abundant quantities of important nutrients. It's vital to get as many nutrients as possible from fresh foods and to use supplements only to fill in the minor blanks in your diet. The following Supplement Protocols are designed for metabolic enhancement, diabetes management, and support for treatment of diabetic complications. For information about specially formulated, blood type–specific supplements, visit our Web site, www.dadamo.com.

Note: If you are taking insulin or diabetes medications, or are being treated for a related condition, consult your doctor before taking any supplements.

Blood Type AB: Pre-Diabetes/ Metabolic Enhancement Protocol

For support of overall metabolic health and blood sugar regulation		
SUPPLEMENT	**ACTION**	**DOSAGE**
High-potency multivitamin, preferably blood type–specific	Nutritional support	As directed
High-potency mineral complex, preferably blood type–specific	Nutritional support	As directed
Larch arabinogalactan	Promotes intestinal health, excellent fiber source	1 tablespoon, twice daily, in juice or water
Probiotic	Promotes intestinal health	1–2 capsules, twice daily
L-carnitine	Promotes metabolic health, energy, active tissue mass	20 mg daily
Holy basil (*Ocimum sanctum*)	Improves stress response	500 mg, 1–2 capsules, twice daily

Blood Type AB: Type 1 Diabetes Adjunct

Add these supplements for type 1 diabetes		
SUPPLEMENT	**ACTION**	**DOSAGE**
Quercetin	Prevents diabetic complications	300–600 mg, twice daily
Zinc	Prevents deficiency common to type 1 diabetics	25 mg daily

Blood Type AB: Type 2 Diabetes Adjunct

Add these supplements for type 2 diabetes		
SUPPLEMENT	**ACTION**	**DOSAGE**
Quercetin	Prevents diabetic complications	300–600 mg, twice daily
Asian ginseng	Stabilizes blood sugar and prevents post-meal hyperglycemia	100–300 mg, 40 minutes before eating (avoid if you have high blood pressure)

Blood Type AB: Diabetic Complications Adjunct

Add these supplements, as appropriate, to support treatment for diabetic complications		
SUPPLEMENT	**ACTION**	**DOSAGE**
Gotu Kola (*Centella asiatica*)	Improves circulation, promotes wound healing, lowers blood pressure	100 mg, 1–2 capsules, twice daily (do not take if you are pregnant)
Vitamin E	Acts as an antioxidant and promotes healing	400 iu daily
Evening primrose oil	Improves nerve function and relieves symptoms of diabetic neuropathy	6 grams daily for 6 months

SUPPLEMENT	ACTION	DOSAGE
Dandelion (*Taraxacum officinale*)	Reduces edema	250 mg capsule daily, or fresh in salad or tea
Stinging nettle root (*Urtica dioica*)	Reduces edema	500 mg, 1–2 times daily, away from meals

The Exercise Component

BLOOD TYPE AB is a true enigma, with the digestive tract and circulatory system of A, the immune system of B, and the stress response of O. Thus, you require both calming activities and more intense physical exercise. Vary your routine to include a mix of the following—two days calming, two days aerobic.

Calming

Hatha yoga: Hatha yoga has become increasingly popular in Western countries as a method for coping with stress, and in my experience it is an excellent form of exercise for Blood Type AB. Make sure that you spend plenty of time outdoors: The effects of sunlight and fresh air work marvels at revitalizing your endocrine and immune systems.

Aerobic/Weight-Bearing

Any of the following can be useful to round out your fitness regimen.

EXERCISE	DURATION	FREQUENCY
Aerobics	45–60 minutes	2–3 x week
Martial arts	30–60 minutes	3 x week
Cycling	45–60 minutes	3 x week
Hiking	30–60 minutes	3 x week
Weight lifting	30 minutes	2 x week

Getting Started: The First Month

IF YOU ARE NEW to the Blood Type Diet and exercise plan, the following guidelines will introduce you to the Blood Type AB regimen over a period of one month. Follow these recommendations as closely as possible, using a journal to record your personal experience with the diet. In addition to measurable factors, such as weight loss, blood sugar regulation, and blood pressure, take the time to note changes in energy levels, sleep patterns, mood, and overall well-being. Over time you'll learn to manage your diet and exercise patterns to achieve the maximum results.

Blood Type AB Diabetes Diet Checklist

Derive your protein primarily from sources other than red meat. ☐ Low levels of hydrochloric acid and intestinal alkaline phosphatase make it difficult for Type AB to digest, and can create a range of metabolic problems. Soy products and seafood are your best choices. Include regular portions of richly oiled cold-water fish. Fish oils can boost your metabolism.

Include modest amounts of cultured dairy foods in your diet, ☐ but avoid fresh milk products, which cause excess mucus production.

Smaller, more frequent meals will counteract digestive problems caused by low stomach acid. Your stomach initiates the digestive process with a combination of digestive secretions and the muscular contractions that mix food with them. When you have low levels of digestive secretions, food tends to stay in the stomach longer.

You'll digest and metabolize foods more efficiently if you avoid ☐ eating starches and proteins at the same meal. The use of digestive bitters 30 minutes prior to a meal can also help you digest foods more efficiently.

Eat lots of BENEFICIAL fruits and vegetables. ☐

Avoid caffeine and alcohol (except red wine), especially when ☐ you're in stressful situations.

Don't undereat or skip meals. Eat blood type–appropriate snacks ☐ between meals if you get hungry. Avoid low-calorie diets. Remember, food deprivation is a huge stressor. It raises stress hormone levels, lowers metabolism, encourages fat storage, and depletes healthy muscle mass.

Week 1

Blood Type Diet and Supplements

- Eliminate your most harmful AVOID foods—chicken and corn. These foods seriously interfere with proper metabolism.

- Include your most important BENEFICIAL foods at least 5 times this week.

- Incorporate at least one SUPER BENEFICIAL food into your daily diet. For example, have a handful of peanuts as a snack, or toss some fresh pineapple and cherries over your morning cereal.

- Eat some cultured soy (miso, tempeh) every day.

- Drink 2 to 3 cups high-quality green tea every day. (My favorite is Itaru's Premium Green Tea, which is available from our Web site.)

- To improve blood sugar regulation, eat 5 to 6 small meals throughout the day, rather than 3 large meals.

- If you haven't already done so, find out your secretor status (see Appendix B to order the test). If you're a non-secretor, increase your compliance by making the recommended adjustments in your diet.

Exercise Regimen

- Plan to exercise at least 4 days this week, for 45 minutes each day.
  2 days: aerobics and weights
  2 days: yoga or T'ai Chi

- Use your journal to detail the time, activity, distance, and amount of weight. Note the repetitions used for each exercise.

▪ WEEK 1 SUCCESS STRATEGY ▪

Start slowly, giving yourself a chance to get used to the Blood Type AB Diet. You'll have a much better chance of long-term success if you take some time to incorporate the Blood Type Diet recommendations into your daily life. I've found that the biggest indicator of failure is a rigid adherence to the plan from the first day on. I know you want to get moving and start seeing results. That's a positive goal. But patience is your friend if you want to make a permanent change in your diet and lifestyle.

Week 2

Blood Type Diet and Supplements

- Begin to eliminate the next level of AVOID foods—beans and legumes.
- Eat at least one BENEFICIAL animal protein every day. Experiment with using very small quantities of meat and BENEFICIAL seafoods, mixed with tofu and vegetables.
- Continue to incorporate SUPER BENEFICIAL foods into your daily diet.
- Continue to eat 5 to 6 small meals throughout the day, rather than 3 large meals.
- Choose the NEUTRAL foods listed as "Allowed Frequently" over those listed as "Allowed Infrequently."

Exercise Regimen

- Continue to exercise at least 4 days this week, for 45 minutes each day.
  2 days: walking or light aerobic activity
  2 days: yoga or tai chi
- If your work is sedentary, get in the habit of taking a couple of "movement" breaks during the day. Walk around the block or up and down stairs.

▪ WEEK 2 SUCCESS STRATEGY ▪

Don't leave home without a quick energy snack tucked into your purse or briefcase.

- Super Smoothie in a Thermos, made with 1 tablespoon whey-based protein powder blended with 1 kiwi, ½ cup pineapple juice, and 1 peeled papaya
- Trail mix: peanuts, walnuts, dried cranberries, dried cherries

Week 3

Blood Type Diet and Supplements

- When you plan your meals for week 3, choose BENEFICIAL foods to replace NEUTRAL foods whenever possible. For example, choose tofu over chicken, or kiwi over a peach.

- Eliminate all remaining AVOID foods.

- Liberally incorporate SUPER BENEFICIAL foods into your daily diet.

- Completely wean yourself from coffee, substituting Itaru's Premium Green Tea.

- Continue to eat 5 to 6 small meals throughout the day, rather than 3 large meals.

Exercise Regimen

- Continue to exercise at least 4 days this week, for 45 minutes each day.
  2 days: walking or light aerobic activity
  2 days: yoga or T'ai Chi

- Add one day of unstructured exercise—walking, biking, swimming.

▪ WEEK 3 SUCCESS STRATEGY▪

Make your meals times of relaxation, not anxiety. Always eat sitting down, avoid stressful discussions, and chew each bite slowly, putting down your fork between bites.

Week 4

Blood Type Diet

- Continue at the week 3 level, focusing on BENEFICIAL and SUPER BENEFICIAL foods.

- Continue to eat 5 to 6 small meals throughout the day, rather than 3 large meals.

Exercise Regimen

- Continue at the week 3 level.

- Evaluate your progress, referring to your journal. Determine which exercise regimen has worked for you, including time of day, setting, and activity level. Look for ways to improve your performance and endurance.

■ WEEK 4 SUCCESS STRATEGY ■

Combat exercise boredom:

- Find an exercise buddy. A brisk morning walk with a friend can reinvigorate your daily effort.
- Cross-train. Choose a different aerobic activity every day.
- Challenge yourself with specific goals: time, endurance, pace. Reward yourself when you reach your goals.
- Don't overtrain. It can cause injuries and blood sugar imbalances.

FAQs: Blood Type AB and Diabetes

Can I use the glycemic index on the Blood Type Diet?

The glycemic index measures the amount of carbohydrates in foods. However, it is not *how much* carbohydrate, but *what kind* of carbohydrate, that makes the difference. The glycemic index is only one aspect of food analysis. The Blood Type Diet goes beyond the general observation of a food's effect on blood sugar levels, evaluating the kinds of sugars present, any lectin activity, the relative amount of beneficial substances, and other blood type–specific issues. For instance, pineapple juice contains anti-inflammatory and protein-digestive enzymes. Black cherries are an important source of antioxidants. To avoid conflicting information, stick with your blood type food list. It takes all of your health needs into account.

I have constant sugar cravings, even when I stick closely to the diet for Blood Type AB. Any suggestions?

Very often this type of sugar reaction complicates an otherwise nice result from the diet. Usually it's just that the liver is having some problems adjusting to the new way of eating and needs some rehabilitation. Try taking the herb milk thistle for a few weeks and drink a cup of licorice root tea at about 10:00 A.M. and 2:00 P.M. (Do not use licorice without physician supervision if you suffer from high blood pressure. In that case, substitute deglycyrrizinated licorice—DGL—which is safe for hypertensives.)

A Final Word

IN SUMMARY, the secret to fighting diabetes with the Blood Type AB diet involves:

1. Increasing active tissue mass (calorie-burning tissue) by eating a diet rich in soy protein, healthy seafood, minimal meat, and green vegetables.
2. Minimizing consumption of the insulin-mimicking lectins so abundant in AVOID beans, grains, and vegetables that are not recommended for your blood type.
3. Improving your metabolic health, lowering your cholesterol, controlling your blood pressure, and lowering your risk for heart disease by limiting high-fat foods.
4. Improving overall metabolic health by engaging in a regular exercise program that includes both aerobic and calming activities.
5. Using supplements intelligently to block the effect of insulin-mimicking lectins, provide antioxidant support, and protect delicate nerve tissue from destruction.

Appendices

A Simple Definition of Terms

agglutination: Clumping, or "gluing" together. One means by which the immune system defends against foreign matter and toxins, notably against lectins and opposing blood type material.

antibody: The product of the immune system when it is stimulated by specific antigens. There are many classes of antibodies, among them "agglutinins," which isolate foreign substances by clumping them together so that they can be eliminated. Blood Types O, A, and B manufacture antibodies to other blood types. Blood Type AB, the universal recipient, manufactures no antibodies to other blood types.

antigen: A chemical that provokes an immune system antibody response. The blood type "ID" present on the blood cells, identified as Type A or B, is one example. A Type AB cell has both of these antigens. The blood type having no antigen is described as O—or

"Zero." As we age, it is to our advantage to shore up our store of circulating anti–blood type antigens, as lower levels mean increased susceptibility to diseases arising from substances and organisms bearing opposing antigens.

biomarker: The biochemical predictor of physiological events (such as cancer or a long life). William Evans and Irwin Rosenberg coined the term to describe those aspects of physical function on which healthier aging particularly depends. Basal metabolic rate (influenced by proportionate muscle mass), aerobic capacity, strength, blood sugar tolerance, body fat percentage, and bone density together provide a reliable indication of one's "biological age," or the health of one's total physical system.

blood type: The term commonly used to refer to the ABO blood group system. Originally used primarily to determine suitable blood and organ donor–recipient matches, ABO type determines many of the digestive and immunological characteristics of the body, as well as susceptibility to the diseases arising from infection, immune suppression, and digestive impairment. It is also one of the tools of anthropology in establishing the origins, socioeconomic development, and movements of ancient peoples.

carbohydrate intolerance: More common in Blood Types O and B, especially non-secretors. A condition in which simple carbohydrate foods such as starch and sugar are not easily or fully digested. Because of the more acidic stomach environment of Blood Types O and B, these carbohydrates remain overlong in the digestive system, leading to a toxic bowel, higher body fat, and prolonged overproduction of insulin and elevated triglycerides. Given sufficient quantities of carbohydrates in the diet, an individual of any blood type can develop this intolerance.

cholesterol: A fatlike steroid alcohol found in animal tissue, especially the brain, nerve fiber sheaths, liver, kidneys, and adrenal glands. Approximately 90 percent of the body's cholesterol is produced by the liver, with the remaining amount obtained from the diet. High blood cholesterol, especially the levels of LDL (low-density lipoprotein) and VLDL (very low-density lipoprotein), is associated most strongly in Blood Types A and AB with the development of heart disease. Studies have found high HDL (high-density lipoprotein) cholesterol levels, regardless of total serum cholesterol, predictive of long life.

high-density lipoprotein (HDL): With LDL and VLDL, responsible for the transport of cholesterol and fats in the bloodstream. HDL is the "good" lipoprotein (fat/protein molecule) of the cholesterol trio. Relatively high HDL levels (over 60 mg/dL) have been correlated with a lower risk for heart disease, especially in women.

hypertension: Persistently high arterial blood pressure, often without noticeable symptoms, a risk factor for the development of heart disease, kidney disease, and stroke. A 140/90 reading is the high pressure threshold for age forty and younger; for those over forty, 160/95.

hyperthyroidism: The overactive thyroid, conventionally treated with long-term antithyroid drugs, surgical removal, or partial removal or destruction with radioactive iodine or surgery. Thyroid diseases show a preference for Blood Type O individuals. While medical intervention is recommended in the case of hyperthyroid function, reducing the types and amount of anti–blood type lectins present in the diet, especially those found in certain grains and legumes, can be of great help in resolving these conditions.

hypoglycemia: Low blood glucose levels. Symptoms include nausea, weakness, dizziness, and cold sweat. Hypoglycemia can be resolved through the use of appropriate protein foods and the avoidance of deleterious lectins, refined starches, and sugar.

hypothyroidism: Underproduction of thyroid hormone thyroxine (t3), and/or free triiodothyronine (t4), conventionally treated by hormone replacement therapy. Thyroid conditions often respond favorably to a blood type–appropriate diet.

insulin: A polypeptide hormone secreted by the beta cells of the islets of Langerhans in the pancreas to reduce high blood sugar levels. Inappropriate diet can trigger defective insulin response, leading to fatigue, overweight, and the development of diabetes mellitus and other metabolic dysfunctions, as well as magnifying the effects of estrogen.

insulin resistance: The condition in which insulinlike lectins, bound to fat molecules' insulin receptors, signal the fat cells to continue to store rather than release the fats for fuel. Triglyceride conversion is impaired, resulting in a sluggish metabolic rate that promotes further fat storage. Non-secretors particularly, and individuals with grain- and sugar-based diets generally, have a greater risk of developing insulin resistance.

intestinal alkaline phosphatase (IAP): An enzyme manufactured in the small intestine, involved in the breakdown of dietary proteins and fats, including cholesterol, and in the assimilation of calcium. In Blood Types O and B, animal protein meals stimulate IAP production levels, thereby lowering blood cholesterol levels and improving calcium absorption. Blood Type O secretors typically have the highest IAP response, followed by Blood Type B secretors. There is evidence that the A antigen possessed by Types A and AB acts to bind, or neutralize, nearly all of the little IAP they produce.

ketosis: A condition marked by a high level of ketones in the urine, produced through a high-protein, low-carbohydrate diet, which forces the body to burn fat for energy. The state of ketosis allowed early humans to maximize their energy, metabolic efficiency, and physical strength. For Blood Type O individuals, maintaining a state of mild ketosis can be key to stabilizing the metabolism and losing weight without sacrificing active tissue mass.

lectins: Proteins that attach to preferred receptors in the human body. Food lectins are often blood type–specific. A lectin's action may initiate agglutination, inflammation, the abnormal proliferation of cells of the immune and nervous systems, or insulin resistance, depending on the type of cells targeted. Abundant in the vegetable kingdom, lectins are fewer in number and type among animal foods, such as eggs, fish, and meats.

low-density lipoprotein (LDL): The "bad" lipoprotein (fat/protein), which acts, with HDL and VLDL, as a carrier for cholesterol and fats in the bloodstream. While small quantities are necessary, less than 100 mg/dL is desirable, 130 to 159 mg/dL is borderline high, and over 160 is a positive risk factor for the development of heart disease and atherosclerosis.

Metabolic Syndrome (formerly Syndrome X): The name given to a cluster of metabolic dysfunctions: insulin resistance and obesity, accompanied by elevated blood-sugar, blood pressure, triglycerides and LDL cholesterol, and low HDL cholesterol. This group of conditions is a precursor to the onset of type 2 diabetes, heart disease, and atherosclerosis.

metabolism: The aggregate of physical and chemical processes by which organisms maintain life, in the opposing functions of building tissue (anabolism) and breaking down tissue and foreign matter to be used as fuel (catabolism).

triglycerides: The body's fat stores, also present in the bloodstream. They are an important source of energy for the heart muscle. Elevated triglycerides are a risk factor for heart disease and stroke, especially in association with high LDL cholesterol and/or insulin resistance.

type 1 diabetes: A condition that occurs when the pancreas is unable to produce insulin. It usually begins in childhood or young adulthood and lasts throughout a diabetic's life. Type 1 accounts for about 10 percent of all diabetes cases.

type 2 diabetes: A condition involving the insufficient production or the poor utilization of insulin, a hormone necessary for the proper utilization of glucose.

very low-density lipoprotein (VLDL): A lipoprotein (fat/protein) substance that carries cholesterol and fats, including triglycerides, through the bloodstream. VLDL is considered the "worst" form of cholesterol, as fairly low amounts are associated with increased risk of heart disease and atherosclerosis.

Resources
and Products

General Diabetes Resources

Organizations

American Diabetes Association
1701 N. Beauregard St.
Alexandria, VA 22311
1-800-DIABETES (1-800-342-2383)
www.diabetes.org
     The nation's leading nonprofit organization for diabetes research, information, and advocacy.

National Institute of Diabetes and Digestive Kidney Diseases
National Institutes of Health
9000 Rockville Pike
Bethesda, MD 20892
301-496-4000
www.niddk.nih.gov

An arm of the NIH that conducts and supports clinical research on the full spectrum of metabolic diseases.

Diabetes Research Institute
University of Miami School of Medicine
1450 N.W. 10th Ave.
Miami, FL 33136
305-243-5300
www.drinet.org
An international center dedicated to the cure and treatment of diabetes.

Children with Diabetes
www.childrenwithdiabetes.com
An online community for kids and families. This is an excellent resource for all diabetes-related issues and concerns.

Nutrition Research
The Institute for Human Individuality
Southwest College of Naturopathic Medicine
2140 E. Broadway Road
Tempe, AZ 85282
480-858-9100
www.ifhi-online.org
The Institute for Human Individuality is under the 501c3 status of Southwest College of Naturopathic Medicine. Its prime goal is to foster research in the expanding area of human nutrigenomics. Nutrigenomics seeks to provide a molecular understanding for how common dietary chemicals affect health by altering the expression or structure of an individual's genetic makeup.

Products
Diabetes maintenance requires a variety of products, including blood glucose meters, injection products, insulin, insulin pumps, and meal-planning aids. An excellent, comprehensive product database is available at www.childrenwithdiabetes.com.

Blood Type–Specific Resources

Dr. Peter D'Adamo

Dr. Peter D'Adamo and his staff continue to accept new patients on a limited basis. To find out more about scheduling an appointment, please contact:

> **The D'Adamo Clinic**
> 2009 Summer St.
> Stamford, CT 06905
> 203-348-4800

www.dadamo.com
The World Wide Web has proven to be a valuable venue for exploring and applying the tenets of the Blood Type Diet and lifestyle. Since January 1997, hundreds of thousands have visited the site to participate in the ABO chat groups, peruse the scientific archives, share experiences and recipes, and learn more about the science of blood type.

Blood Type Specialty Products and Supplements

North American Pharmacal, Inc., is the official distributor of Blood Type Diet® Specialty Products. The product line includes a home blood-typing kit, the secretor test, books, educational materials, supplements, teas, and support materials that have been specially designed to address the unique requirements of each blood type.

> **North American Pharmacal, Inc.**
> 12 High St.
> Norwalk, CT 06851
> Tel: 203-866-7664
> Fax: 203-838-4066
> Toll free: 877-ABO TYPE (877-226-8973)
> www.4yourtype.com

To purchase supplements mentioned in this book or suggested by your naturopathic physician, your local health-food store is always an excellent resource.

Home Blood Typing Kits

North American Pharmacal, Inc. is the official distributor of Home Blood Type Testing Kits. Each kit costs $9.95, plus $6.50 for shipping and handling, and is a single-use disposable educational device capable of determining one individual's ABO and rhesus blood type. Results are obtained within about four to five minutes. If you have several friends or family members who need to learn their blood type, you will need to order a separate home blood-typing kit for each individual.

The Blood Type Library

The following books are available in bookstores, health-food stores, selected grocery and specialty stores, on the Web, and through North American Pharmacal.

Eat Right 4 Your Type: The Individualized Diet Solution to Staying Healthy, Living Longer, and Achieving Your Ideal Weight
Dr. Peter J. D'Adamo, with Catherine Whitney
G. P. Putnam's Sons, 1996
The original Blood Type Diet® book, with over two million copies sold in more than sixty-five languages.

Cook Right 4 Your Type: The Practical Kitchen Companion to Eat Right 4 Your Type
Dr. Peter J. D'Adamo, with Catherine Whitney
G. P. Putnam's Sons, 1999 (Berkley Trade Paperback, 2000)
Includes over 200 original recipes, thirty-day meal plans, and guidelines for each blood type.

Live Right 4 Your Type: The Individualized Prescription for Maximizing Health, Metabolism, and Vitality in Every Stage of Your Life

Dr. Peter J. D'Adamo, with Catherine Whitney
G. P. Putnam's Sons, 2001

Eat Right 4 Your Type Complete Blood Type Encyclopedia
Dr. Peter J. D'Adamo, with Catherine Whitney
Riverhead Books, 2002

The A-to-Z reference guide for the blood type connection to symptoms, diseases, conditions, medications, vitamins, supplements, herbs, and food.

4 Your Type Pocket Guides: Blood Type, Food, Beverage, and Supplement Lists
Dr. Peter J. D'Adamo, with Catherine Whitney
Berkley Books, 2002

The Eat Right 4 Your Type Portable and Personal Blood Type Guides are pocket-sized and user-friendly. They serve as a handy reference tool while shopping, cooking, and eating out. Each book contains the food, beverage, and supplement list for each blood type plus handy tips and ideas for incorporating the Blood Type Diet into your daily life.

Eat Right 4 Your Baby: The Individualized Guide to Fertility and Maximum Health During Pregnancy, Nursing and Your Baby's First Year
Dr. Peter J. D'Adamo, with Catherine Whitney
G. P. Putnam's Sons, 2003

An invaluable guide for couples looking to combine the best of naturopathic and blood type science to improve the health of mother and baby—with practical blood type–specific guidelines for achieving maximum fitness before pregnancy, eating and living right during pregnancy, and how to continue in good health during Baby's first year.

Index